MORE
Spiritua

D0809014

"Our memories are stor͏e[...] [...]n
they are memories of peace, love, and healing, what we give
birth to is a gift to the parents and the world. As a father of
five, I know from my wife's experience that the contents of
this book speak the truth."

—Bernie Siegel, MD, author of *Love, Magic
& Mudpies* and *Prescriptions for Living*

"The mother-infant bond is one of the most intimate,
powerful connections that exists, and it begins long before
birth. *Spiritual Pregnancy* is the best guide I know on
developing, nourishing, and sustaining this blessed state.
This book raises the pregnancy literature to a new level."

—Larry Dossey, MD, author of *Healing
Words* and *The Power of Premonitions*

"For all those who see pregnancy as a spiritual journey, as
well as parents-to-be seeking a closer connection to their
unborn child, doctors Shawn Tassone and Katie Landherr
lay out the way. Expert integrative obstetricians, they guide
you through the traditions of the ancients and illuminate
the vibrant path to your own hero's journey."

—Victoria Maizes, MD, executive director
of Arizona Center for Integrative Medicine;
professor of medicine, family medicine,
and public health; co-author of *Be Fruitful:
The Essential Guide to Maximizing Fertility
and Giving Birth to a Healthy Child*

"Doctors Shawn Tassone and Kathryn Landherr have used their extensive experience in obstetrics and integrative medicine to invite you to explore the deeply intuitive nature of pregnancy and the magic and wonder of birth. From the practical to the profound, I'm confident you will find what you are looking for within this book's pages. I highly recommend it."

—Tieraona Low Dog, MD, fellowship
director at University of Arizona
Center for Integrative Medicine

"*Spiritual Pregnancy* does an incredible job at marrying the physical and the spiritual, the medical and psychological, and even Western and Non-Western approaches. It is a caring, insightful, and obstetrically smart look at one of the most miraculous physiologic events there is. It will be a great resource to anyone having a baby, and it makes me proud to be an ob-gyn. Well done!"

—Jennifer Ashton, MD, leading
medical correspondent for ABC
and ob-gyn physician

Spiritual
PREGNANCY

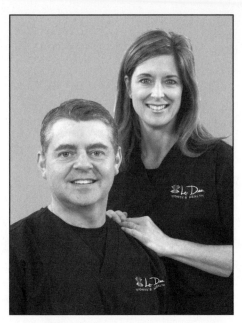

About the Authors

Shawn A. Tassone and Kathryn M. Landherr are board-certified obstetrician gynecologists practicing in Austin, Texas. As a unique team of married physicians, they bring a rare perspective to the topic of women's health. Kathryn is a graduate of the University of Texas and completed her medical training at Texas A&M Scott and White Hospital. Shawn attended Regis College and completed his medical training at the Creighton University School of Medicine. They both finished residency at the University of Oklahoma Health Sciences Center. Visit them online at http://aaobgyn.com.

They have worked with medical luminaries Andrew Weil, Jon Kabat-Zinn, James Gordon, and Larry Dossey, and are considered international experts in mind-body medicine, integrative medicine, and spirituality in health. They have lectured internationally on topics of menopause and bioidentical hormones, spirituality and pregnancy, indigenous healing practices, mind-body medicine and women's health, and integrative medicine, and they are the first scholars to bring the work of Joseph Campbell and the hero's journey and superimpose it over pregnancy, the ultimate hero's journey.

Spiritual PREGNANCY

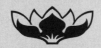

Develop, Nurture
& Embrace
the Journey
to Motherhood

Shawn A. Tassone, MD
and Kathryn M. Landherr, MD

Llewellyn Publications
WOODBURY, MINNESOTA

FIRST EDITION
First Printing, 2014

Author and yoga pose photos by Anne Daiva Photography
Cover design by Gavin Duffy
Cover photo: iStockphoto.com/Aldo Murillo
Interior lotus glyph from Fleurons of Hope font
Interior journaling cue image from *1167 Decorative Cuts
CD-ROM and Book* (Dover, 2007)

Llewellyn Publications is a registered trademark
of Llewellyn Worldwide Ltd.

Cover model used for illustrative purposes only
and may not endorse or represent the book's subject.

Library of Congress Cataloging-in-Publication Data
Tassone, Shawn A., 1967–
   Spiritual pregnancy : develop, nurture & embrace the journey to motherhood / Shawn A. Tassone, MD, and Kathryn M. Landherr, MD. —First edition.
      pages   cm
   Includes bibliographical references.
   ISBN 978-0-7387-3551-1
   1. Pregnancy—Popular works. 2. Mind and body—Popular works. 3. Motherhood—Popular works. I. Landherr, Kathryn M., 1966– II. Title.
   RG551.T38 2014
   618.2—dc23
                                                              2014029883

Llewellyn Worldwide Ltd. does not participate in, endorse, or have any authority or responsibility concerning private business transactions between our authors and the public.
   All mail addressed to the author is forwarded, but the publisher cannot, unless specifically instructed by the author, give out an address or phone number.
   Any Internet references contained in this work are current at publication time, but the publisher cannot guarantee that a specific location will continue to be maintained. Please refer to the publisher's website for links to authors' websites and other sources.

Llewellyn Publications
A Division of Llewellyn Worldwide Ltd.
2143 Wooddale Drive
Woodbury, MN 55125-2989
www.llewellyn.com
Printed in the United States of America

To our parents,
where our spiritual journeys began.

To our children,
where our spiritual journeys were renewed.

Medical Note

Please note that the information in this book is not meant to diagnose, treat, prescribe, or substitute consultation with a licensed healthcare professional. Both the authors and the publisher recommend that you consult your medical practitioner before attempting the techniques outlined in this book.

Contents

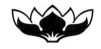

Contents

Journeywork Exercises

Yoga Poses

Acknowledgments

Writing a book is akin to giving birth. This book gestated for close to two years and would not have been born without the tenacity of our agent and midwife Katharine Sands of the Sarah Jane Freymann Literary Agency. We thank Katharine for her faith in us and for her vision for our books and writing in the future. Katharine is a true champion. We would like to thank Llewellyn Worldwide Publications and Angela Wix for believing in this project and the mysticism of pregnancy; we hope to have a long and happy relationship with you.

To Toni Robino and Doug Wagner of Windword Literary Services: thank you for literally being our heroes. We're amazed by how you magically spun straw into gold and wove it together to create the book we envisioned. You are true professionals, and it's been a joy to work with you.

To Lauren Summers: thank you for vetting our spiritual and cultural material, smoothing out some of our raw material, and blessing us with your support. Thank you to Barbara Barnett, Pandora Peoples, Nina Amir, and Phoebe Collins for your spiritual and cultural contributions to this book. As talented writers who understand the hero's journey through a unique connection to spirit, your words speak volumes to the hearts of our readers. To Barbara, thank you also for your generous contribution to the "Life after Birth" chapter. Thank you to Gretchen Kelly for adding ideas and content from your world travels.

Our deepest gratitude goes to Jennifer (Wolfe) More, the prenatal yoga teacher and doula who brought the powerful influence of yoga to this project. Jennifer has many DVDs on Prenatal Vinyasa Yoga, and she tours the world training yoga teachers and doulas and teaching women how to care for their babies through the power of yoga. All of the pictures and explanations of yoga postures are from Ms. More.

Finally, we want to thank our patients. Accompanying these women warriors on their hero's journey of pregnancy is what inspired us to write this book. Mothers are the true warriors of our race; without them, we would not only cease to be, we also would lose all connection to the sacred.

Foreword

If you have picked up this book, you are probably about to embark on one of the most transformative journeys of your life: the journey of becoming a parent. And luckily for you, you have stumbled onto two of the most knowledgeable guides who exist in this field: Shawn Tassone and Kathryn Landherr. With their combined experience of more than thirty years of serving mothers-to-be as ob-gyns, they offer a vast amount of medical expertise and first-hand experience that will support you in making a safe passage on this journey.

There are several things that you need to know as you set off on this great life adventure, the first being that your life will be changed forever—and for the better. This transformative experience is a fascinating process that has captivated all cultures throughout recorded history. Some experts, including Joseph Campbell, believe that the process of transformation has a recognizable pattern for all human beings—beginning with a calling and preparation, followed by crossing thresholds and finding treasures, and ending with the realization that you are no longer the same being who started on the journey.

In my research and practice, I have studied the process of transformation extensively. I have found that there are several things that are crucial to the success of growth and transformation.

Firstly, it is important to have a support system in place to help you get clarity about your experience and prevent you from feeling lonely, overwhelmed, or disconnected. Your support network will provide you with companionship, resources, inspiration, guidance, connection, and stability during the difficult parts of transformation. In addition, research shows that supportive relationships have beneficial effects on the cardiovascular, endocrine, and immune systems of the body. Another essential ingredient to your success is the ability to be still, listen deeply, and see the interconnectedness of everything. Yoga and meditation are great tools to help you achieve this goal. Once you delve into the depths of yoga and meditation, you will find a world most easily described as "energy." Concepts of energy (also known as qi, chi, or prana) can be found in Eastern cultures from the past five thousand years. Energy is the life force that is part of everything that exists and that sustains living beings. The more you practice yoga and meditation, the more you will be able not only to experience this energy but also to transform it.

With the guidance of Dr. Tassone and Dr. Landherr, you will learn to practice yoga, meditation, and much, much more so that you can navigate this process of transformation in a smooth and graceful way. Not unlike the caterpillar becoming a butterfly, the expecting mother engages in a remarkable development that changes all aspects of physical form and consciousness. May your journey of becoming this new being be blessed. May the longtime sun shine upon you, all love surround you, and the pure light within you guide your way on.

Sat Nam.

Gabrielle Pelicci

Gabrielle Pelicci, PhD, is a certified Kundalini Yoga instructor, massage therapist, and Healing Touch practitioner. She maintains a private practice in holistic health in Los Angeles, Miami, Philadelphia, and Washington, D.C. Gabrielle has also traveled to twenty countries in Asia, Africa, South America, and Europe to study different cultural approaches to healing. She is the author of *Portraits of Her: A Narrative Analysis of the Life Stories of Five Women Healers*.

Introduction

Spiritual Pregnancy maps out the path that we wish all women had the opportunity to follow as they prepare for motherhood. As ob-gyns who have assisted in bringing hundreds of children into the world and who have four children of our own, we're inspired to share what we've learned and serve as your guides during this life-altering experience.

We believe that carrying a baby and giving birth awaken and deepen a woman's connection with earth, god, goddess, and all that exists in the tangible world of the senses and the intangible world of the soul. If ever there were an epic hero's journey, this is it. During the next nine months, your strength and your resolve will be tested. You will experience discomfort, anxiety, and fear as you stride forward into unknown territory. But you will also discover that you're stronger, wiser, and braver than you thought you were. You will experience joyful bliss, eager excitement, and moments of speechless awe. And you will experience a new level of connection with other mothers in your life, including those who came before you. But, most profoundly, you will get in touch with the voice of your own soul. And while we wrote this book from our frame of reference as husband and wife, the message applies to a broad range of pregnancy experiences, including single mothers and gay couples.

When we told some of our friends and a few patients at La Dea Women's Health that we were working on this book, they all thought it sounded great. But when we told our colleagues, some of the reactions were mixed. Some thought it was a good idea; others asked why "serious medical doctors" were dabbling in the spiritual domain. The answer is simple: for us, spirituality and medicine go hand in hand.

Both of our medical careers have traditional beginnings, with Shawn earning his MD at Creighton University and Katie earning her MD from Texas A&M. We both completed our residencies in obstetrics and gynecology at the University of Oklahoma Health Sciences Center, where Shawn was the administrative chief resident. But our education didn't end there. As practicing doctors, we both continued our education and our inspired missions to broaden and deepen our understanding of health and healing.

Consequently, as an associate fellow in integrative medicine at the University of Arizona under Andrew Weil, Katie is well versed in all aspects of health and healing, including mind and body connections and spirituality.

As a fellow of integrative medicine also under Andrew Weil at the University of Arizona, Shawn is knowledgeable about many forms of healing used not just in this culture, but also in ancient and modern cultures around the globe. Shawn's five years of doctoral study in mind-body medicine and nonlocal healing have convinced him that there is more to pregnancy and birth than meet the eye. On his journey to better understand the fullness of life and health, he has spent time with John of God (a medium and psychic surgeon in Brazil), Huichol shamans, and Peruvian healers. This and the work of Rick Strassman, author of *The Spirit Molecule: A Doctor's Revolutionary Research into the Biology of Near-Death and Mystical Experiences,* have deepened our appreciation of and respect for the spiritual side of life. Strassman's work draws a potential link between chemicals the birthing mother produces and her ability to transcend space-time as she delivers her baby from the internal world of her womb to the external world.

We have also both studied and learned about the healing aspects of breathwork, or *pranayama*—the extension of the life force through breathing. On that path we learned of the many benefits yoga has as a health practice for mind, body, and spirit. We feel that yoga is a vital part of a spiritual pregnancy and enjoyed consulting with renowned yoga expert Gabrielle Pelicci in selecting the poses to include for each trimester and birth. Our first book, *Hands Off My Belly: The Pregnant Woman's Survival Guide to Myths, Mothers, and Moods,* introduced women to the physical aspects of pregnancy and giving birth. This book immerses you in the spiritual world of pregnancy and birth.

Your Epic Journey

You'll soon discover firsthand that this journey is as much about your transformation to motherhood as it is about being pregnant and birthing your baby. That's why our guidance is illustrated with the stories of our patients, friends, and family members who have made this journey. (To respect the privacy of the moms, dads, and their babies—many of whom are now teenagers—we changed their names and identifiable information.) We've also included stories, information, legends, and lore from a variety of cultures and spiritual traditions so you can see how your journey is similar to and different from mothers around the world, from ancient times to modern. To offer you a broad spectrum of spiritual perspectives, we've also included appendices of contributions from Nina Amir, Barbara Barnett, Phoebe Collins, and Pandora Peoples.

To provide you with the best step-by-step guidance possible, we've divided the book into five parts that are organized by the three trimesters, birthing, and beyond. Each part of the book includes journaling cues as well as spiritual exercises called journeywork that will support your personal transformation, reduce stress, and give you an opportunity to connect with the guidance and love of your soul and also with your baby and their soul.

At the end of parts 1–4 we offer yoga poses that we selected based on Katie's experience and Jennifer (Wolfe) More's guidance (http://www.prenatalvinyasayoga.com/). Jennifer is a registered Yoga Alliance vinyasa and prenatal yoga instructor, doula, childbirth educator, reiki master, and mother. We highly recommend that you take the time to learn and practice these poses. If you have any concerns about practicing them, please check with your physician first.

We encourage you to create a computer file or buy a lovely notebook and colorful pens—or both—to chart the course of your spiritual pregnancy. You can use your "journey book" to do the written journeywork exercises, respond to the journaling cues in each chapter, and record your yoga practice, nutrition, hours of sleep, or anything that you choose to closely observe and document over the next nine months.

In part 1, the first trimester, your journey begins with your call to adventure: discovering that you're pregnant. We walk you through your first trimester physically and spiritually. You'll learn how to begin bonding with your baby, why it's important to strengthen the love bridge with your mate, and you'll also select "mother mentors" from your friends and family and from the spiritual realm.

Part 2 is the oasis in the middle of your pregnancy: the second trimester. During the second trimester your body is starting to blossom with the radiance of hosting a new life, and soon you will feel baby move, stretch, or kick. This thrilling moment, called the quickening, awakens a new reality about your role as mother. This is when you may begin questioning the parenting advice you've heard or read and looking deeper into your own mind and heart for the answers you seek. The journeywork, journaling, and yoga in this part of the book are designed to make you more flexible and resilient both physically and emotionally. You'll be strengthening your physical and spiritual arms and legs for the next part of the journey—and beginning to sprout your wings.

Part 3 supports you during the final months of your pregnancy: the third trimester. Here you will be learning how to turn challenge into change as you gain more confidence in yourself and prepare for birthing your child. You'll also find out how to help establish sleeping patterns for your baby while you're still pregnant; connect more deeply with your baby and your own spiritual power by working with the elements of earth, fire, air, and water; and emotionally ready yourself for the physical separation with your baby that will occur at birth.

Part 4 guides you through the rite of passage of birthing—whether the event takes place at home with a midwife or in the hospital. You'll discover that both experiences are rich with opportunities for spiritual awakening, bliss, and magic. This is the point in the journey where everything you've learned over the past nine months culminates to support you in successfully bringing your baby into the world.

Part 5 will assist you in reentering your "ordinary world" as a new person with a new identity and a new child. Sometimes called "the resurrection" in a hero's journey, the exercises in this part of the book will assist you in making your way back home and back into your community as a changed woman with a sacred, living Grail.

If you're in your second or third trimester, begin the book with part 2 (second trimester) or 3 (third trimester) so that you're reading what's most pertinent to where you are now and what's coming up. Then go back and read the earlier parts in the book, too, because there's important information, introspection, and yoga poses that we don't want you to miss.

Ready or not, the journey has begun…

Spiritual Pregnancy: The Hero's Journey

As with all epic journeys, your pregnancy is an opportunity for you to grow and blossom physically, mentally, and spiritually. Here is a summary of some of the highlights that await you:

The Ordinary World: This is the world you live in before your epic journey begins.

The Call to Transformation: You discover you're pregnant and are called to the journey toward motherhood. Even if part of you wants to remain in the safety and comfort of your ordinary world, the call beckons you forward. The call to adventure makes your goal clear: to carry and birth a healthy baby. It also sets the stakes for your journey; achieving your goal is largely up to you. In symbolic terms, your goal is to offer a divine and Holy Grail to the world, or a new spirit in physical form.

Reluctance: No matter how much you thought you wanted a baby, the reality may raise doubts or fears. This is normal and expected. The secret here is to amplify the voices of your heart and soul and drown out the inner critics.

Wisdom and Mentors: Women you know (and some that you don't know) appear in your life to offer assistance and guidance. This is also a time in your journey to reach out to mother-mentors whom you admire. Watch them. What secrets can you glean? Ask them. Listen carefully to the pearls of wisdom they offer. And since this is a spiritual journey, this is also the time to connect with the divinity within yourself and your own wise inner voice. You may discover that communing with one or more "mother goddesses" in the spirit realm can bring you insights, peace, and confidence. This stage of your journey is also about learning how to ask for help. If you were in a small village, all of the women would know you are pregnant, and many would take it upon themselves to pitch in where they noticed that you needed help. Since you are probably not living in that type of environment, honor the other women in your life by calling upon them to assist you. This is a gift for them as much as it is a help to you.

Crossing the First Threshold: When you move from the first trimester into the second, you are crossing the first threshold. You have become accustomed to the idea of being pregnant, and you fully enter the world of motherhood by agreeing to face the challenges that lie ahead. For many women, the moment they feel the baby move for the first time is also the moment they symbolically cross this threshold. You officially leave the old world— and the old you—behind and embrace the path to motherhood.

The Initiation: An epic journey wouldn't be epic were it not for the tests, difficulties, and woes that must be faced and surmounted along the way. This stage of your journey, during the middle part of your pregnancy, is a time for emotional and spiritual transformation as your body physically transforms. This is when the hero begins to learn the rules for this extraordinary world and encounters new challenges. This might mean getting real with yourself about your diet and nutrition choices, giving up a little fun to get more sleep, or healing emotional wounds that you don't want to carry with you into motherhood. It might also mean making amends with estranged family members, rethinking parenting methods, and agreeing to disagree about an issue that you and your partner vehemently disagree about. Motherhood is filled with making compromises, and this is a good time to get better at that.

Approaching the Inmost Cave: As you enter the last three months of your pregnancy, you, as the hero, are approaching the inmost cave. On this journey that cave is the physical and spiritual womb, where the reward of your journey awaits you. It's natural for the hero to experience some anxiety and fear during this approach; your life is about to change dramatically. But by this point on your journey, your unconditional love for your baby is so deeply entrenched that you are willing to do whatever it takes to meet them. As your labor begins, your body lets you know that you have just a little more time to center yourself and prepare for the "ordeal" ahead.

The Ordeal: While the word *ordeal* has a negative connotation, the event itself actually holds the potential for a positive outcome. On your journey, birthing is considered the ordeal because it is the most physically and emotionally challenging part of your journey. This is where you stand in all of your strength and bring everything that you've learned on this journey to the table, figuratively and sometimes literally. During a movie, this is a moment of tension and suspense as we hold our breaths for the best outcome.

The Reward: Your eyes behold your beloved baby—the Holy Grail—for the first time, and your heart soars with a level of joyful bliss that only a mother knows. You have triumphed in your goal to bring this new spirit safely into the world, and your heart sings as your partner and all of your loved ones celebrate this miraculous event with you.

The Road Back: During the days following the birth, you and your baby make your way back to the "ordinary world" where you will build a life together. It's important to be gentle with yourself during this time. Being a supermom is different from being a superwoman. Don't try to do everything that you can by yourself. Gift your family members and loved ones with the opportunity to serve you as you acclimate to active motherhood.

Resurrection: You feel fully awake, alive, and well again. You're energized and ready to let some of your helpers go as you adjust to the changes that baby has brought into your daily life. You know you have been changed and transformed by the birth of your baby, and you know that much more transformation lies ahead. While birth is the culmination of your pregnancy journey, it is also the beginning of your parenting journey, and there is always much to learn.

Returning with the Reward: Your new baby is ready to be introduced to your relatives, friends, and coworkers. They are the physical manifestation of the spiritual intention that was sparked prior to your pregnancy, and now you are sharing this treasure with others.

Part 1
First Trimester

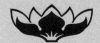

Crossing the First Threshold

Congratulations! You're officially on your way to motherhood. You are about to embark on a spiritual journey complete with all the highs and lows and thrills and chills. We guarantee that it will all be worth it. The path from conception to birthing and beyond is an epic journey with you in the leading role as hero. And keeping in sync with the classic "hero's journey," once you conceive and a new life begins taking shape inside of you, your heart, mind, and spirit become a matrix of change. You are the very embodiment of the place of transformation between worlds: between the world of the unborn and the born. From out of the void of potential energy, a spark of life has been ignited that shines within your womb.

Your developing baby connects you to generations past—parents to grandparents to great-grandparents. No matter your family's traditions or cultures, your baby connects you to the history and legend of antiquity, forming an unbreakable link from generation to generation. Procreation permeates holy texts in most traditions. Passing on the teachings, history, traditions, and rituals is both a religious and a cultural imperative—a sacred obligation—

and so the welcoming of a new life into the family is steeped in customs that may be centuries old.

The new spirit and developing baby also connect you and your partner to the Divine—the creator of all things, God and Goddess. Parents are the spiritual bridge between humanity and divinity. As your pregnancy takes root within your womb and the first inklings of *really* having a baby begin to dance in your imagination, you begin to change inside. Cells are dividing and growing within you as you form the organ that will nourish your child for the next nine months.

In our modern culture, we often neglect the inner life of the expectant mother and her baby and concentrate on the physical. Examinations and ultrasounds are par for the pregnancy course, but the more subtle emotional and spiritual aspects of this most marvelous time of life are often ignored. As ob-gyns who are married to one another and who have raised four of our own children, we believe that body, mind, and spirit are equal partners in the pregnancy journey. A totally aware pregnancy is a successful pregnancy. A spiritual pregnancy is, in essence, a mindful pregnancy. This approach offers a path along which you transform your own spirit as you bond with the spirit of your baby. While your body is preparing to give birth to a new life, you are preparing to give birth to a new you.

And so begins your epic journey.

First Trimester:
What's Happening?

Month One
Physically

- Your partner's sperm meets your egg, and fertilization occurs.

- Once fertilized, the egg nestles into the nourishing lining of your uterus.

- Your hormones surge, and the baby and the placenta begin to develop.

- By the end of this month, the baby, though small as a grain of rice, begins to take shape.

Spiritually

At the same time that egg and sperm meet, your spiritual essence combines with your partner's in the act of conception. Energy, matter, and spirit join together, and a new life begins. No matter how scientific we are about conception, there will always be an element of mystery and magic. For example, doctors can't explain why, but many women say they have a sense of being pregnant just moments (or a day or two) after they have conceived. Whether you know you're pregnant during the first month or not, your life force is interacting with the new life that is growing inside of you.

Month Two
Physically

- The baby is about the size of a pea.

- The baby's heart is divided into two chambers and beats 120 to 160 times every minute.

- Every minute, about one hundred thousand nerve cells are being created.

- All the internal organs are formed.

- By the end of the month, the baby is about an inch long and is starting to move.

Spiritually

As your heartbeat increases by about fifteen beats per minute and the baby's heart beats almost twice as fast as your own, you are poised to experience a "spiritual quickening," or what might be called a stirring of spirit. Some women say that, for no apparent reason, they start feeling more spiritual, closer to God/Goddess, and at peace with themselves and the world at large. During this time it's not unusual to experience a surge in your passion for life. You may also experience a deep inspiration for serving your purpose, which includes loving and caring for the new being that your body, mind, and spirit is nurturing.

Month Three

Physically

- The baby is transforming from an embryo to a fetus resembling a miniature human being.

- The baby's teeth, tongue, and vocal cords begin to form, and they can open and close their mouth, swallow, and even hiccup.

- The baby starts to grow fingernails and toenails, can move the arms and legs, and can open and close their hands.

- The baby's genitalia differentiate into male or female; by the end of the month, an ultrasound can often reveal the baby's gender.

- By the end of the first trimester, the baby is about 2.5 to 3 inches long and weighs about an ounce.

Spiritually

As your awareness of the new life inside of you grows, you will likely find yourself pondering the mysteries of life: Who am I? Where do I come from? Where am I going? Why am I here? Even if you've had clear answers for those questions in the past, your spiritual pregnancy may prompt you to revisit them. These are good questions to ponder while practicing yoga, meditating, and journaling.

Chapter 1

The Birth of a Mother

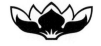

*A journey of a thousand miles
begins with a single step.*
Confucius

A mother is born in small steps day by day, over time, just like her baby. Perhaps your journey toward motherhood began when you were a child, feeding a dolly and pretending to be a mother—or maybe it wasn't until you finally met "the one" and found yourself daydreaming of rocking a baby to sleep. You may have been trying to conceive for years and spent a small fortune in fertility drugs. Or maybe you didn't think much about becoming a mother until you saw the little white strip turn blue.

The journey begins differently for each woman and each pregnancy. But what all pregnant women have in common is the epic journey toward birth—a journey that is filled with great adventure and that profoundly changes you and your world. Whether this is your first pregnancy or your fourth, you are standing on the threshold to growth, transformation, and communion with the Divine. In a real sense, pregnancy is a hero's journey: a quest that can make you stronger, wiser, and more spiritually awake. As a hero on a spiritual journey, you're not only preparing to give birth to a child, you're also preparing to give birth to a mother. When you think of yourself in this role, what traits come to mind? Are there mothers whom you admire and wish to emulate? What characterizes the mothers whom you *don't* want to model? These are a few of the questions that will help shape your spiritual pregnancy because the answers reveal your own soul's highest values.

Robin Lim, midwife and founder of Yayasan Bumi Sehat (Healthy Mother Earth Foundation)—which offers medical aid, free prenatal care, and birthing services to any woman who needs it—says, "Birthing is the most profound initiation to spirituality a woman can have."[1] In motherhood, mothers emulate creation. And Barbara Katz Rothman, author of *Re-creating Motherhood,* says, "Birth is not only about making babies. Birth is about making mothers—strong, competent, capable mothers who trust themselves and know their inner strength."[2]

As a woman on this journey of inner and outer transformation, you are a matrix of power with the potential for involution and evolution. You are the fulcrum of psychological, spiritual, and physical change, the ultimate manifestation of potential.

The power of producing new life has been considered mystical and sacred around the world throughout time. Artistic depictions of women ripe with child can be found on every continent and in most faiths. In African literature and culture, motherhood is a sacred and powerful spiritual component of a woman's life. In Mexican culture, motherhood is intrinsically related to spirituality.[3] All around the world, throughout history, there are depictions of mother goddesses.

One reason that motherhood has been revered in many cultures is the belief that women who are pregnant can walk between the worlds of physical and spiritual, seen and unseen. The shamanistic culture of Siberia has a saying that a woman is, by her nature, a shaman. What they're saying is that women can walk with one foot in the physical world and one foot in the spiritual, and we believe that this may be especially pronounced during pregnancy and childbirth. When your menstrual blood flow abates and life begins within, the membrane between worlds seems to become thinner and more translucent. During this time you and the baby are on journeys with the same sacred purpose: life. This heightened awareness occurs in tandem with physiological changes in both you and the baby, and it is sometimes referred to as a spiritual quickening.

The Call to Transformation

All great journeys begin with a call that, if heeded, is sure to change you. In literature and legend this call often comes in the form of otherworldly signs or messengers. The hero receives messages from the world beyond that something big is going to happen, and she's going to be at the center of it.

In the story of the birth of Buddha, for instance, Queen Maya, Buddha's mother, went to bed in the middle of a midsummer festival. She left the festivities and fell into a deep sleep. In her slumber, she dreamt that a beautiful white bull elephant walked around her three times with a white lotus in his trunk. He tapped her on the side with his trunk and then vanished into her. Wise men were brought to interpret the dream, which they said meant that Maya would bear a son. If this son left the royal family, he would become a Buddha, or an enlightened being. There are many illustrations of this marvelous beginning to Buddha's life, showing the beautiful Maya receiving her dream of giving birth to him.

Another compelling image of the call to transformation is Botticelli's *Annunciation*. It depicts the moment when the angel Gabriel appears to Mary to announce that, although she is a virgin, she is to bear the child Jesus. When Mary hears this, her body sways like a flower in an invisible breeze, parting her dark cloak to reveal a pink dress that may symbolize eternal innocence. Leaning toward Gabriel, she seems to be beckoning at the same time her hand gestures appear to be holding him at bay. In this image, Mary illustrates the combination of awe and apprehension that typically characterize the call to the spiritual journey of motherhood.

Though the journey toward motherhood begins at different times for different women, the journey of motherhood begins at conception for all women. The awareness that you're pregnant calls you to transform physically and spiritually. On a hero's journey this is sometimes referred to as the call to adventure. You're standing on a threshold that leads to a new way of life for you and a new life on the planet. In his famous essays on the hero's journey, Joseph Campbell calls the moment when the hero is invited to step over the threshold to begin the journey "the call."[4] And the call is not always easy to heed. Accepting the call means accepting transformation. Whatever may lie ahead, you're agreeing to do your part to bring this new life safely into the world. At the moment that you consciously accept this call, you cross the threshold, and your new life as a mother begins.

 . . . .

Journaling Cue: Take a few moments to write about your thoughts and feelings when you first discovered you were pregnant. How do those thoughts and feelings compare with what you are thinking and feeling now?

It takes courage, strength, and a strong sense of purpose to accept the call. If it didn't, it wouldn't be a hero's journey. In the sections of the Christian Bible from which the "Hail Mary" prayer comes, the angel Gabriel says to Mary, "Blessed art thou among women, and blessed is the fruit of thy womb." Mary is at the threshold. She breathes deeply and then answers the angel that she is indeed ready to accept the gift of the child in her womb. In the story of the Buddha, Queen Maya receives the dreams that tell her she will bear a magical child, the Buddha. She accepts the interpretation of the dream and her destiny as a new mother. The threshold has been crossed. The divine mother has been born.

The Sacred Womb

Like Mary and Queen Maya, you have a physical womb—your uterus—and you have an energy center behind your uterus that is sometimes called a spiritual womb. Located just behind your uterus, your spiritual womb is also the general location of your womb chakra, also called the sacral chakra. Chakras are areas of your body where you collect and store energy. The concept of chakras has ancient roots in both Hinduism and Buddhism. Each of the primary chakras corresponds to particular systems and organs in our bodies. Your womb chakra corresponds to your reproductive system, liver, and bladder. This energy center is associated with creativity, sensuality, and unadulterated sexual pleasure. Psychologically, the womb chakra corresponds with relationships, pleasure, emotional needs, enthusiasm, and joy. In Celtic thought, the womb chakra is likened to the cauldron from which divine beings bring creation. As your body ripens with new life, the womb chakra pulses with energy that feeds the divine transformation that is beginning to occur.

We've both seen physical manifestations of the power of the chakra system, especially in the sacral, or womb, chakra. One of the most dramatic was Kelly, our patient who was six months pregnant and experiencing excruciating pain in her pelvis. Her x-rays and blood work indicated that everything was in working order, so Shawn gently asked her if she'd had any recent relationship issues. She burst out crying. Her husband had just admitted that he was having an affair. As soon as he confessed his infidelity, Kelly began remembering being raped when she was eighteen. She had repressed the traumatic event for many years, but her husband's devastating news had ripped the scab from the wound. After talking with her, her pain began to ease, but she was still in a good bit of discomfort. Shawn referred her to an empathetic psychologist for emotional therapy. When she returned two weeks later, her pain had lessened significantly. While the affair was not an event she would have wished for, she was able to see that it helped to expose an older wound and give her the opportunity to heal it. Her therapist was helping her to face and work through the fear and anger blocking her sacral chakra and causing her real physical pain.

Journeywork
Warming the Womb Chakra

Reserve thirty to forty-five minutes to sit quietly and allow your consciousness to sink into your womb chakra. You may want to light a candle or dab a scented essential oil onto your belly. Choose a scent that smells ripe and sensual such as jasmine, sandalwood, or musk.

Inhale and exhale slowly and deeply. Focus on your abdomen expanding and contracting with each breath.

When you begin to feel relaxed and present, close your eyes.

Visualize the inside of your womb glowing with a warm reddish-gold light like the embers of a fire. With each inhalation, see the embers glowing more brightly until they look like a small fire or a miniature sun. This is the vibrant, creative, and nurturing energy of the womb chakra. Imagine you can feel the pleasant warmth gently infusing the walls of your womb with physical strength. Imagine your baby's spirit inside this tiny sun, being fortified and enriched with sacred light.

Allow the warmth of this energy and the vibrancy of your baby's spirit to spread through your entire abdomen, up through your chest and down through your hips. See the light expanding as it envelops you from head to toe, relaxing every muscle in your body and vanquishing any feelings of anxiety or worry that you may have.

Bask in this warm, safe place for as long as you like.

When you're ready, ask your baby if they have a message for you.

Listen carefully so you can accurately write this message down in your journey book. The message might come to you in the way of words, images, or sensations. There are no right or wrong messages. The meanings of some messages will be obvious immediately, while others may not become clear until later in your journey. If you feel as though you have not received a message directly from your baby, write down the thoughts that crossed your mind during this journey. It's best to write the message or thoughts in your journey book before speaking to anyone.

Welcoming a New Spirit

When the spirit or soul enters the human body is a long-debated issue. Many traditions state that this occurs at the quickening, or the time when the mother begins to feel the baby's movements in utero. For most women this doesn't occur until the second trimester, around the seventeenth to twentieth week. Whatever your beliefs, there is a chemical process that begins in the fetus around weeks seven to nine when the pineal gland is formed.

The pineal gland has been referred to as the "third eye" in many mystical traditions, so it's no shock to discover the location of this gland is the center of the brain. It is thought to produce melatonin, a very powerful hormone and antioxidant that controls our sleep and wake cycles. Rick Strassman has speculated that the pineal gland might also be where a compound called dimethyltryptamine (DMT) is produced. DMT is a naturally occurring hallucinogen that may be released at times of intense stress such as death, near death, birth, and episodes of intense or severe pain.[5]

In Strassman's work *DMT: The Spirit Molecule,* he discusses the theory of DMT and the pineal gland being visualized in the human body at the forty-ninth day of fetal development.[6] In the Tibetan Book of the Dead, there's a description of the reincarnation process and how after death the soul undergoes a forty-nine-day spiritual journey toward rebirth. One can see the potential here for information coming from the mystical traditional of Buddhism and the scientific materialism of Western research. If the spirit is looking to enter or reenter the body forty-nine days after death, and DMT (the spirit molecule) begins production in the human body around the forty-ninth day in utero, maybe we should consider looking into this synchronicity with more observation and an open mind. Around the forty-ninth day of fetal development, we recommend that you foster a receptive state of mind. The following journeywork will support you in achieving and maintaining a welcoming vibration.

Journeywork
Preparation for the Forty-Ninth Day

Journal daily and pay special attention to synchronicities or coincidences; also record your dreams for later interpretation. Try not to wait to record dreams; when you wake, jot them down in your journey book before going back to sleep. Spend more time in meditative practice, possibly ten to fifteen minutes per day, and with your inhalations and exhalations focus on the baby inside you and surround them with that welcoming love that only a mother can provide.

Opening to Mother-Mentors

In world myths, legends, and fairy tales about the hero's journey, the first part of the pilgrimage is usually punctuated by the arrival of a spiritual ally or mentor. This mentor will guide the hero through trials and tribulations toward the ultimate goal. In *Cinderella*, for instance, the mentor is the fairy godmother. In world cultures such as the Native American Navajo, spiritual mentors often take the shape of humble insects or animals. The Navajo's Spider Woman, for instance, is a strong spiritual ally and guide for women in childbirth. She is often seen in the shape of a spider as she spins the web of existence into being.

Spiders also figure in the theme of the ancient Minoan goddess Ariadne, who in later Greek myth helped the hero Theseus out of the labyrinth with the help of a golden thread (or web). In pre-Greek times, Ariadne was a goddess in her own right. She was the goddess of the labyrinth and also a guide and mentor for women in all stages of sexuality, including childbirth. Ariadne's origin as a prepatriarchal goddess of the labyrinth shows her connection with the womb (the labyrinth was an ancient metaphor and symbol for the womb). Like Ariadne, the Navajo Spider Woman weaves connections between the worlds of the born and the unborn and the past, present, and future. Both these traditional spiritual mentors are loving and wise guardians of women and of childbirth.

During your hero's journey, once you accept the call to transform, you energetically invite mentoring from other mothers—both physical and spiritual. The mentors you choose in the physical realm will be the women you most cherish in your life: perhaps your own mother or a close friend or relative whose parenting you admire. And you don't have to venture far from your hearth to find them. The sisters, mothers, and grandmothers who you enjoy sharing a hot cup of tea with in your kitchen often make the best mother-mentors for your spiritual pregnancy. The practice of older women passing wisdom down to their daughters, granddaughters, nieces, and friends is as old as humanity itself.

 . . . .

> **Journaling Cue:** In your journey book, write a
> description of your ideal mother-mentor. Do not
> censor yourself as you include all the traits and
> qualities that this ideal mother-mentor would
> have. Next, make a list of women you know who
> demonstrate the traits and qualities on your list.
> Consider which women you might like to invite to
> be allies on your journey.

Journeywork
Choosing Your Mother-Mentors

Joseph Campbell described the mentors on the hero's journey as "the benign, protecting power of destiny…a reassurance—a promise that the peace of Paradise, which was known first within the mother womb, is not to be lost…One has only to know and to trust and the ageless guardians will appear."[7] Your mother-mentors may include not only the physical guardians whom you listed previously but also guardians and mentors from the spiritual realm.

Your background and beliefs will guide you in selecting the spiritual mentors who are perfect for you. Perhaps you resonate with Ariadne or you may gravitate to the Navajo Spider Woman. Kwan Yin, the Buddhist bodhisattva (enlightened being), is thought to be the goddess of compassion. She hears the cries of the world and is also the protector of women. All these spiritual mentors are wise guardians of women and childbirth, and with a little research on your own, you can come up with many others to choose from. The most important thing to remember is that the mentors on this journey are yours to choose, and the team you assemble will be the perfect team for you and for your baby, even if you don't consciously know why you have chosen all of them. You can select from the mentors we introduce here and in the following Essential Elements section, or you can explore various mother goddesses from around the world in order to find your own. But there's no need to make this complicated. It's perfectly fine to choose one or more mother figures whom you're already familiar with from your own religion or sacred tradition.

 . . . .

Journaling Cue: Once you've chosen your spiritual mentor or mentors, write their names and a little about them in your journey book.

Essential Elements and Associated Mentors

The miracle of life requires the essence of four of the earth's primary elements: fire, water, earth, and air. During your pregnancy, these elements all play a part in nourishing and sustaining both you and your baby. Each element is associated with spiritual mother-mentors from a variety of world cultures.

Fire

Your spiritual pregnancy begins with the spark of life at conception. Throughout human history, people have honored fire and considered it sacred. In Ireland, for instance, Saint Brigid was originally Brigid, the goddess of fire, smithcraft, and creativity. Throughout Ireland there are many holy wells associated with Brigid. For centuries, women visited these wells to tie wishing rags on the nearby tree branches for health and safety in childbirth and for the healthy future of their unborn children. Before Saint Patrick and others brought Christianity to Ireland, there was an important home shrine to the goddess Brigid where nineteen nuns kept a sacred flame burning for her. Today, a small order of nuns continue the tradition in Kildare and dedicate the eternal flame to peace and reconciliation in the world.

In traditional Chinese medicine, fire is the element associated with blood, circulation, and the heart. Throughout your pregnancy, the circulation in your lower extremities may be weaker, causing swelling and fatigue. During your nine-month journey, it's important to temper this fire so that it is warm but not hot. The meditations and yoga poses throughout the book will help you to do this.

Water

Water is the element most associated with birth and rebirth. Used in spiritual rituals throughout the world, water is cleansing, soothing, and purifying. Up to 60 percent of your body is composed of water, and the amniotic fluid that protects your baby is mostly water. In a sense, we carry the sea in our veins. Celebrated for its life-giving properties, water can renew and refresh our bodies and our souls.

One of the most renowned spiritual mother-mentors associated with water is Yemanja, a deity originally of the Yoruba religion that originated in Africa. A dark-haired beauty often depicted rising out of the sea, Yemanja is the essence of motherhood and the guardian of children. She is often referred to as the mother of all mothers. There are many regional variations on this orisha's name. In Africa she is known as Yemoja and Mami Wata; in Haiti she is called La Sirene (the mermaid); and in the Dominican Republic she is known as Yemalla or La Diosa del Mar (Sea Goddess). In the United States she is called Yemalla, Yemana, and Yemoja.[8]

In traditional Chinese medicine, water is associated with your kidneys and bladder. Keeping these organs healthy and strong will make the next eight months more comfortable. During your spiritual pregnancy, the water element is about your courage to adapt to your changing body and changing life. Water shows us how to shapeshift so we can move smoothly around obstacles, and it reminds us to go with the flow.

Earth

Earth is the element most strongly connected with being centered and grounded. We're rooted in the earth and also in the lineage of our ancestors. When you become pregnant, you connect with your ancestral tree right back to the first mother. When Katie was pregnant, she felt stronger and more grounded than she'd ever felt before. This is something we hear from a lot of the mothers we assist.

The earth element is associated with your stomach, spleen, and pancreas. These organs help you to digest your food and provide sustenance for you and baby. On a spiritual level, the earth element is empathy. It empowers you to connect with and care for others, particularly your developing child.

One of the mother-mentors closely associated with the earth element is Ixchel, the ancient Mayan goddess of midwifery and medicine. Early in the sixteenth century, Mayan women traveled to Cozumel to visit the sanctuary of Ixchel and pray for a marriage blessed with children. Ixchel is also a goddess of medicine, herbs, and other remedies from the soil. When you incorporate gentle, physician-approved herbs into your pregnancy, you're following a long line of ancestors who practiced the same earth-centered medicine.[9]

Here are some common herbs that are considered generally safe for women during pregnancy. (**Note:** Be sure to check with your own physician before taking any herbal remedy.)

Alfalfa

This herb is a good source of vitamins and minerals, particularly vitamin K, which is essential for normal blood clotting.

Ginger Root

Sipping an herbal tea made with ginger or sucking on a small slice of the peeled root can help to ease nausea, improve digestion, and aid circulation. There are also some delicious treats made with ginger. Just be aware of the amount of sugar in them, and use them moderately.

Oat Straw

Oat straw has a host of healthy phytochemicals, nutrients including calcium, folate, iron, magnesium, manganese, phosphorus, potassium, selenium, zinc, and vitamins A, B, and E. It acts as a restorative nerve tonic, so it can relieve anxiety and stress and ease insomnia.

Peppermint

Peppermint leaf tea can aid digestion and increase your appetite. Drink it sparingly during your pregnancy, though, because it may interfere with iron absorption. For that reason, avoid it altogether when you're nursing.

Red Raspberry Leaf

Red raspberry leaf tea can enrich mother's milk and help the uterus to contract more effectively. (**Note:** During the first eight months of your pregnancy, do not drink more than one cup of this tea per day because you do not want to encourage contractions during that time.)

Herbs to Avoid

Some herbs should be avoided during pregnancy.

Cleansing herbs that are too strong to use during pregnancy or may be irritating to you or your baby include: arnica, barberry, bee balm, black walnut, blessed thistle, catnip, chaparral, chicory, coltsfoot, comfrey, ephedra, fenugreek, gentian, horehound, horsetail, ipecac, juniper berries, lobelia, Oregon grape root, poke root, rhubarb root, rosemary, uva ursi, and yarrow.

The following herbs should be avoided because they can negatively affect your hormones during pregnancy: borage, damiana, dong quai, licorice, sarsaparilla, and Siberian ginseng.

The following herbs can bring on contractions or bleeding, so they should all be avoided: angelica, birthwort, black cohosh*, blue cohosh*, cotton root, elecampane, fenugreek, feverfew, goldenseal, horehound, lovage, mistletoe, motherwort, mugwort, myrrh, osha, parsley, pennyroyal, rue, sage, tansy, thuja, thyme, turmeric, and wormwood. (*Black cohosh and blue cohosh may be used in the last two weeks of pregnancy, but consult with your physician first.)

Laxative herbs that are too strong to be used during pregnancy include: aloe vera, buckthorn, butternut, and cascara sagrada.

Please use caution when using any herbs during your pregnancy, especially during the first trimester.

Air

Life outside the womb begins with the first breath and ends with the last. Without air, we can't survive more than a few minutes. Spiritually we associate air with inspiration. To inspire literally means to inhale. When we're inspired, we experience a sense of peace and grace. Time stands still, and all is well with the world.

In ancient Greek philosophy and science, air is one of the four classical elements. The divinity associated with the element of air was the primeval goddess Khaos. The ancient Greek word *khaos* literally means the gap or the space between heaven and earth. Khaos is the goddess of fate. She's also the grandmother of darkness and light, or night and day. As a mother-mentor, she can help you unite the opposing emotions that your pregnancy may be triggering. She can also carry messages between the physical world and the spiritual world.

The organs we associate with air are the lungs. By taking time each day to center yourself by breathing slowly, deeply, and rhythmically, you can increase your sense of inner peace and connect with the inspiration of your soul.

There's no need to wait until you've selected all of your mother-mentors to move on to chapter 2. As you discover more about spiritually bonding with your baby in the next chapter, they may request a particular mother-mentor or influence your decision through a dream, a gut feeling, or a flash of intuition.

Journeywork
The Breath of Life

Sit on your yoga mat or in a chair that allows you to comfortably sit upright with good posture.

Rest your hands on your thighs, and close your eyes.

Inhale for seven seconds and exhale for seven seconds, silently counting so that your inhalation and exhalation are equal in duration. (If seven seconds feels too long or too short, adjust the time for yourself. Take a deep breath, counting until your lungs are completely expanded. Now take the same amount of time to exhale.)

Continue your balanced breathing for three to five minutes.

Keep your focus on your counting and breathing, allowing other thoughts to drift through and out of your mind. If significant thoughts or feelings arise, record them in your journey book.

Spiritual Lovemaking

Now that you and your partner have created a baby together, you share a new spiritual bond. It is a bond that began with your souls, opened your hearts, and encouraged you to trust each other, see each other more deeply, and love each other more divinely. The spiritual intention to create life opens you to a different dimension of sexual intimacy. Making love with the spiritual understanding that you would feel blessed by conceiving creates a deeper tenderness for each other and solidifies your heart-and-soul connection. Whether you physically conceived your child together or you conceived through other measures, the spiritual intent to bring forth a new life was present in your lovemaking. In essence, energy precedes matter, so you conceived your baby spiritually before you became pregnant physically.

Lovemaking—not just sexually, but also by gazing into each other's eyes, caring for one another, being kind and respectful, and sharing joy, laughter, sorrow, and tears—led to your parenthood. We encourage you to faithfully strengthen your roles as lovers and friends even as you take on the new roles of mommy and daddy. Now is the perfect time to worship each other's divinity, and sharing sexual pleasure is one way to do that. While there are myths that it is unsafe to have sex during pregnancy, modern science has proven otherwise, except in the cases of high-risk pregnancies.

Sex is the language of lovers. But if your breasts are tender, you're exhausted, and nausea has become a way of life, your libido may be hard to find—even if his has kicked into overdrive. Instead of letting this become a point of contention, we suggest a skin-to-skin compromise with no expectation or pressure to do anything but lie or cuddle together. If you find that this sometimes sparks a desire for something more, go with it. If not, enjoy whatever does feel good. There's no doubt that maintaining your intimacy and sexual passion can take some patience and effort during this hormonal transformation, but it's worth it. And during this trimester, when you're feeling up for it, you still have the freedom to enjoy all positions and most of whatever you've been doing up to this point.

Couples who have more than one baby tend to learn this the first time and do what they can to take advantage of these relatively "free-for-all" months. The exception is if you're in a high-risk pregnancy and your physician advises you to abstain from intercourse, orgasm, or both. If you're not at risk, you still should put away any toys that are designed to penetrate your vagina or rectum because these can increase your risk of infection. If you have questions or concerns, please ask your physician. While the Internet can be a wonderful place to find answers, it's also fraught with myths and misinformation.

Science has proven what human beings already knew: that touch is healing. Being touched, hugged, and stroked decreases stress and anxiety. In your fingertips, hands, and arms, you and your partner have the power to help each other and your developing baby to stay healthy and strong. Skin-to-skin sensual touching is soothing in and of itself, and it's also a gentle gateway to lovemaking.

Bonding sexually with your partner is also a great way to help them stay connected to your ever-changing body and the important role that they are playing in the pregnancy. Some partners feel left out and isolated during this time, and they can also feel helpless since it's clear that you're doing all the baby-making work. Having an opportunity to help you slow down and relax and give you sexual pleasure may make you both happier now than it ever has before, and this will give you great joy and power on your hero's journey.

Dispelling Pregnancy Myths

What would an epic journey be without myths and legends? There have always been mysteries in life that humans try to solve with logic and science, and pregnancy and birth are among the most magical of these mysteries. If you were trying to get pregnant, you may have heard advice to lay a baby on your bed, douche with apple cider, let the light of the full moon shine on your belly before making love, and even swallow a watermelon seed. While we don't believe that any of these approaches is the magic elixir of pregnancy, we do believe that your clear spiritual intention can empower any approach. Hippocrates, the father of medicine, was onto something when he theorized that a fetus was the fruit that grew as a result of the joining of the female and male seeds. Aristotle, on the other hand, said, "The woman functions only as a receptacle, the child being formed exclusively by means of the sperm."[10] For a smart guy, he was way off on that one.

Once humans discovered how conception actually occurred, the advice for pregnant women ranged from creative to absurd. Soranus of Ephesus, considered the father of gynecology, said that a woman should rub her belly with the oil of fresh olives after intercourse and refrain from bathing for seven days. He also cautioned women wanting to conceive to avoid rocking chairs. Other doctors advised women to lie on their backs with their legs tightly crossed.[11] If a woman missed her menses, Pliny the Elder said she should drink a concoction made from the ashes of a porcupine and apply a light ointment made from hedgehog fat on her belly. This was supposed to prevent miscarriage.[12]

One of the greatest debates concerning conception surrounded the question of a woman's pleasure. In the thirteenth century, Saint Thomas Aquinas condemned the idea of a woman actually enjoying intercourse, but other theologians argued that a woman's pleasure played a part in the beauty of the baby. Later in the same century, men were advised to prolong their lovemaking until their wives climaxed. They were assured that this practice would give them the best chance of producing a healthy, aesthetically pleasing baby.[13]

In the Middle Ages, the bellies of pregnant women were thought to be filled with mysteries and magic and were sometimes feared by men. Pregnancy was alternately considered to be some sort of illness, especially if a woman was thought to be carrying a girl. Nearly everyone on record agreed that during pregnancy women should abstain from sexual intercourse. One of the few physicians to take a stand against this in the seventeenth century was a doctor named Dionis. He went out on a limb by admonishing his colleague Mauriceau for prescribing abstinence. Dionis said, "Mauriceau could not have made these observations at firsthand, having never had a single child in forty-six years of marriage. For me, who had a wife who became pregnant twenty times and gave me twenty children that she successfully brought to term, I am persuaded that the husband's caresses spoilt nothing."[14] Good for Dionus! And thank goodness for a voice of true experience.

As you walk this path, whether for the first time or the fifth, you will appreciate the voices of experience, and your inner voice will guide you toward the mentors and support that you desire. Your sacred womb will blossom energetically even as it slowly expands physically, and you will begin to tune in not only to the voice of your own soul but also to the silent voice of your unborn child. As transcendent as this spiritual communion is, it's equally important for you to stay physically centered and grounded. Working with the elements in the exercises we introduced in this chapter and staying open to the guidance of your spiritual mother-mentors as well as the wise women in your daily life will keep you strong, healthy, and vibrant throughout this journey.

Chapter 2

Bonding Before Birth

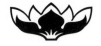

The life of a mother is the life of a child: you are two blossoms on a single branch.
Karen Maezen Miller,
Momma Zen

Zoe ran her hands over her slightly rounded belly as she smiled and said, "It's like we already sort of know each other." Zoe was referring to the baby she was carrying. In the first trimester, the emotional bond many women feel with their babies can best be described as surreal. The awareness that you're hosting a new life, a precious little being, is with you at all times. And this awareness alone can begin to create a bond between you and your baby long before they are born.

Each woman's connection with her developing baby is unique, but all women light up when they talk about it. For some women, the hero's journey really takes off when they realize that their baby responds to them. "When I sing to her, she wiggles around," said

Diana, who was well into her second trimester. "I love knowing that she knows I'm her mom."

We love hearing mothers talk about this bond, and over the years it's become clear to us that the bonding mothers and fathers do with their babies in utero not only makes them happy, it also lowers stress and promotes a sense of well-being for parents and child.

The Silent Conversation Between You and Baby

There is a silent conversation born from the physical fusion between you and your baby during pregnancy—an unspoken communication that deepens as you journey together toward birth. This two-way communication is conducted with feelings, thoughts, and physical sensations. As you and baby grow together, you each have an innate desire to assimilate with one another. This urge is hard-wired into both brains and encouraged by hormones such as oxytocin, often called the cuddle hormone.

We have seen the deep connection and communication of mother and child before birth on a physical and also what some might call a metaphysical level. For instance, our patient Monica, who was close to full term, was troubled because she was having recurring dreams her baby was suffocating. She felt sure that something was wrong. We sent her to a woman's center, where a non-stress test of the baby showed placental insufficiency—which meant that the child was conserving energy and was indeed suffocating though lack of in utero nutrients. The baby was born healthy via C-section because her mother's intuition urged her to remember the message in her dreams and tell us about it so we could help her.

World culture is rich with strange and wonderful stories of babies communicating with their mothers before birth. In the New Testament it is said that St. John the Baptist "leapt for joy" in the womb of his mother, Elizabeth, when Mary and her unborn child arrived to visit them. In the West African epic *Sunjata,* from the ancient kingdom of Mali, the hero Sunjata occasionally escapes from his mother's womb to play around the house in spirit before birth. When he's ready to be born, he speaks to his mother aloud and tells her so. And in the Kabbalah, the mystery cult of Judaism, it is said that the child in the womb knows everything that God knows. Upon birth, an angel presses his finger to the child's lips to silence him—hence the mysterious indent we all carry over our lips.

But no matter what beliefs you have about the spiritual aspects of pregnancy and childbirth, there are certain physiological processes occurring in your body that are common for all pregnant women. In addition to your body producing hormones such as oxytocin that can calm you and the baby, your body also produces stimulating hormones such as cortisol when you're stressed or angry, and these hormones can have a negative effect on the baby. A recent study reported by Britain's *Guardian* concluded that cortisol in an expectant mother could lead to impaired growth, fatigue, and even depression for her fetus.[15, 16]

Professor Vivette Glover at Imperial College in London and Dr. Pampa Sarkar of Wexham Park Hospital in Berkshire took a blood sample from 267 mothers and a sample from the amniotic fluid surrounding their babies. The report of the experiment published in the journal *Clinical Endocrinology* revealed that at seventeen weeks or older, the higher the cortisol in the mother's blood, the greater the cortisol in the baby's amniotic fluid.[17] Cortisol is a hormone produced by stress, and while it helps to compensate when the body is in crisis, high levels can add to depression, fatigue, and impaired growth. This type of research, along with our own observations from thirty-plus years of combined experience guiding women along this journey, has us convinced that the more emotionally balanced expectant mothers are, the better off their babies will be.

Fortunately, stress hormones are something you *can* control. You can use balanced breathing, meditation, yoga, and the journeywork offered in this book to lower your stress and avoid infusing your bloodstream—and that of your child—with an abundance of stress chemicals. Believe us when we say that doing this is every bit as important as refraining from smoking, drinking, and other unhealthy lifestyle choices.

Studies done in the early 1990s demonstrated that fetuses growing in women suffering from anxiety tended to be more active than fetuses with mothers who did not report anxiety. This prenatal influence was carried into the neonatal period after birth. If the mother's emotions can affect the emotions of her unborn baby, then we think it's feasible for emotions to be imprinted too. That makes us theorize that there may be a prenatal imprinting of personality. While maternal emotions and stress have been shown to influence the prenatal environment, occasional life stresses are normal and may help to make the baby more resilient to stress. We worry more about pregnant women who are in ongoing difficult situations.

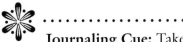

Journaling Cue: Take a few moments to write down your three biggest stresses, and write a little about each one. Why is this making you so stressed out? What is the outcome you wish for in the stressful matter? What can you change or do differently to move closer to the outcome that you desire? You may not have all the answers, but taking worries and fears and exposing them to the light of day takes away some of the power they have over us.

Rest assured that there is solace even for those who are chronically stressed. The baby still garners much comfort in your simple heartbeat and by your ability to take slow, long, deep breaths. If you're feeling overtly stressed, try the following exercise. It will bring your breathing to a point where you can deepen and slow your heart rate, and your infant will follow your lead.

Journeywork
Slow Down, Baby

In this exercise you're stimulating the vagus nerve, which passes through the neck and thorax to the abdomen and the parasympathetic nervous system. This will slow your heart rate and induce a state of relaxation. This is very good for you and your baby.

Inhale deeply while silently counting from one to eight (about eight seconds).

Exhale fully while silently counting from eight to one (about eight seconds).

Repeat this sequence ten times.

Journeywork
Opening the Golden Channel
of Communication

Meditation helps reduce your stress and also your baby's. Even if you've never meditated or had trouble with it in the past, when you do it with the intention to spiritually connect with your baby, it can quickly become your favorite part of the day.

This meditation practice was designed to strengthen the two-way communication between you and your baby before birth. Over time, it will bring the two of you into a more synchronous heartbeat pattern. By the second month of your pregnancy, your baby's heart rate is faster than yours, and it will continue to speed up until the tenth week of your pregnancy, when it starts to slow down. So you won't be trying to match your baby's heartbeat in this meditation; rather, you'll be synchronizing *your* heartbeat pattern with your baby's. That pattern is called a sinusoidal wave. When you inhale, your heart rate goes up. When you exhale, it goes down. The sinusoidal waves are the rising and falling wave patterns that stimulate your nervous system and help to balance your emotions, which is good for you and for the baby.

Since we're doctors, we want to give you the science behind this meditation, but don't let it intimidate you. This meditation is easier to do than it is to explain. This practice's objective is to align your sinusoidal wave pattern with your baby's. If you were doing this with a biofeedback monitor measuring heart rate variability, you'd see your waves rising and falling at the same time.

We believe this synchrony is one of the best ways to share spiritual communion with your developing baby.

You can do this meditation anywhere that's warm and comfortable. If you have a practice of sitting meditation using a firm pillow, that may be your most comfortable position. But if not, try a cushioned chair, your bed, or a warm bath. Try it different places, and find the ones that feel the best to you. We suggest that you record the following instructions using a calm and soothing voice. From about the middle of your fifth month of pregnancy, the baby can hear your voice. But before then, we believe babies can hear their mother's silent intentions.

As I close my eyes, I turn my attention inward to my heart and the heart of my baby. I take full breaths, inhaling through my nose, filling my lungs to capacity, and gently exhaling through my nose until my lungs are empty. As I focus on my breath, I feel the tension leaving my body with each exhalation. With each inhalation, I feel myself and my baby being nourished by the oxygen in the air. I feel my jaw and neck relaxing, and I continue taking full breaths as the sense of relaxation moves down to my shoulders, my back, and my hips. With each full breath, my tension decreases until my entire body feels relaxed and light.

Keeping my eyes closed, I use my inner eyes to see the beating heart of my baby. (If you know your baby's name, use it here.) I see my baby's heart glowing like the embers of a fire. As I inhale, I envision the breath of life fanning the embers of my baby's heart. I feel this warm energy filling my belly and helping me to relax even more. With each breath I see the red glow expand until it touches my heart and fills my chest. I feel my heart open with love for my baby as I envision our wave patterns rising and falling together, maintaining a rhythm that is unique to us. With my inner eyes I can see the waves rising and falling with each slow, full breath. With my heart I can feel the unique rhythm of two hearts beating.

Now, take a minute to speak from your heart to your baby's heart, saying whatever you wish to communicate. After you've finished sharing, continue taking full breaths. Open your heart to the message that your baby has for you. Write your message and baby's message in your journey book.

Sharing Your World with Baby

You are your baby's connection to the outside world. As such, you're the sight, hearing, taste, smell, and touch for them. What your eyes see can stimulate the production of stress or relaxation hormones. What you hear may also be heard by the baby, so enveloping yourself in relaxing sounds also gives the baby a relaxing environment. The food you eat baby eats too, so you have the ability to send a message of caring and love literally with every bite. Certain scents and aromas, such as lavender flowers that encourage you to relax, can have that effect on the baby; so can the stimulating effects of sugar and caffeine.

Your pregnant body is designed to let you know what to avoid. For instance, you may have savored every sip of coffee just a few weeks ago, but now the aroma might make you nauseous. One of our patients who had been a smoker said that the taste of a cigarette was suddenly repulsive. She thought she had the flu, but it turned out that she was pregnant. You may not have sought out the salad bar in days gone by, but now you find yourself craving a calcium-rich spinach salad. The more you listen to what your body truly needs, the more support you'll be giving to the baby.

This is important because not only are the baby's sensory organs growing, so are their brain, pancreas, intestines, nostrils, and lenses of the eyes. Metaphorically, the baby is starting to see their surroundings and digest the meaning of their existence and new life. The baby's understanding of this world begins as they experience your world through your senses, even as development is underway. Toward the end of the third month, hair and nails are growing, and the kidneys are begining to function, thus beginning the production of amniotic fluid.

"Prenates can see, hear, feel, remember, taste, and think before birth," says Luminare Rosen, founder and co-director of the Center for Creative Parenting in Marin and Sonoma counties, California.[18] That means you can commune with your baby through your senses and emotions—and through your dreams, thoughts, and intuition as well. Some doulas and spiritually oriented midwives describe the umbilical cord as a tube of shining golden light. A doula is a trained and experienced professional who provides continuous physical, emotional, and informational support to the mother before, during, and just after birth, or who provides emotional and practical support during the postpartum period. Many midwives and doulas believe this golden light is healing, energizing, and full of positive energy. Holding this image in your mind as you explore various forms of sensory communication with your baby will set your intention to create a loving bond.

For you and your baby, the six senses are the information superhighway of communication, conveying connection back and forth and forging a bond that will last a lifetime. You, as the mother, are the antenna. As such, you'll want to filter out those things you don't wish to transmit and focus on more meaningful messages. Many pregnant women today are working stressful and demanding jobs and have very little downtime. While you may not be able to filter out all of the messages, you can definitely set aside time daily to sit down in a quiet space and send messages to your unborn child. This time allows for unconscious messages to be exchanged between you and baby, and it provides an opportunity for you to assure your baby that they are safe and loved.

 . . . .

Journaling Cue: By spending time each day focusing only on the connection you have with your baby, you can strengthen the lines of communication. Think of a specific message you want to share with your baby, and write that down in your journey book. When possible, share messages that are just one sentence or even one word: *I love you. You are safe. I am joyful.* Or *love, safety, joy.* Listen with your heart, and if you sense that the baby is sending you a message too, write it down.

As a mother in the making, your sensory systems are undergoing changes, and your ability to communicate with your baby through sensory channels is being enhanced. Many women say that their physical senses such as smell and taste are magnified during pregnancy. If a whiff of cigarette smoke used to make your nose wrinkle, now it can make you retch. Even aromas you used to savor, such as bacon and coffee, can go from yum to yuck overnight. And the opposite happens too. Craving olives, ice cream, chocolate, or just plain salt are responses to the physiological and psychological transformation that you and the baby are experiencing. Even your preferences for music, art, literature, and film can change as you and the baby engage in one of the most mystical practices of all time: shapeshifting—not the sci-fi version, but the real thing.

One simple way of showing the effects that the outside world has on an unborn baby is their reaction to a loud or otherwise obnoxious sound. In the OB triage unit when a patient comes in because of decreased fetal movement, we might perform what is called vibroacoustic stimulation testing (VAST). VAST is where a small device is placed against your belly and a buzzing sound stimulates the baby.

In contrast, when the baby is stimulated by loud sounds such as honking car horns, rock concerts, or shouting, there is a discernible increase in heart activity that can be measured. According to Thomas Varney, an expert on the effects of prenatal and early postnatal environment on personality development, prenatal stimulation bodes well for healthy fetal development: "Every minute, there are new brain cells being formed in the unborn child. And as the new brain cells are being formed, pathways or circuits are being formed along the lines that help assist communication for whatever the child needs. For example, the child will obviously need to breathe, the child will need to move when he is born, the eyelids will need to open and close, so all these organs and all the nervous tissue that supply these organs has to start developing long before birth.

"It's the same thing with the brain circuits. The more you stimulate your baby's developing skin by gently pressing on your belly or stimulate their auditory nerves by talking, singing and playing music, the more those pathways develop and become stronger so that when the child is born, they are better prepared for the world." [19, 20] Just avoid loud noises and bangs that can startle the baby and make the heart rate go up.

Touch

With Katie's pregnancies we noticed toward the end of the second trimester that the baby would respond to our touch. A gentle press was often met with a kick or push back from the baby. Most women start to feel their babies move when they're sixteen to eighteen weeks pregnant (more on this in part 2). But you can begin using touch to communicate with your baby as early as you like. You may not be able to feel the baby responding to your touch, but that doesn't mean it's not happening.

When you wash your belly or apply lotion, imagine washing your baby or gently smoothing lotion or their skin. You may want to hum or talk to your baby as you do this, so they connect the sensation of touch with your voice. This is something that your partner can do too. Later in your pregnancy, when you feel your baby's movements, you can communicate even more directly by pressing gently on your belly while talking or singing.

Hearing

Throughout Katie's pregnancies, we both talked to the baby on a daily basis. Before she started showing, people who overheard us probably thought we were crazy. But there's a lot of scientific evidence that indicates babies learn to identify their parents' voices before they're born, and this is something we've known for quite some time. In a 1984 study, French scientists found that babies less than two hours old responded more to their mothers' voices than to the voices of five unfamiliar females.[21] More recent studies show this as well.[22] So if you think babies can't hear or identify voices until *after* they're born, think again.

In a study conducted by Queen's University in 2003, sixty full-term fetuses showed spiked heart rates when their mothers read a passage from a book out loud[23]—so read, sing, chant, and recite nursery rhymes to your baby. Studies have found that children who have been read nursery rhymes in the womb react positively to those rhymes after birth, often responding to them like verbal security blankets. But you don't have to be that formal about your communication; simply talking works great too. Tell your baby how your day is going or what you're making for dinner. Share a favorite memory from your past, such as how you met their father. Talk about your plans for the future—your hopes and dreams. Anything pleasant will do.

Venezuelan clinical psychologist Dr. Beatriz Manrique's classic study on the effect of pre- and postnatal stimulation proved the theory that babies who were stimulated with touch and sound in the womb were more vital and active at birth. The newborns in her control group whose mothers had communicated with them before birth had more developed head control and were able to move their heads in the direction of their parent's voices.[24]

Smell

Smell is the middle child of the senses, but it is the sense that lingers the longest in the brain. Scents can be stimulating, relaxing, invigorating, and soothing. Many aromas from nature captured in essential oils can promote energy, restful sleep, and a sense of well-being. Rose oil, lavender, geranium, and sandalwood all have soothing, calming effects on the nervous system. Citrus, peppermint, and eucalyptus have stimulating effects. And when you experience these effects, so does your baby. Work with an aromatherapist or educate yourself about the effects of various scents so you can choose the best aromas for various situations and circumstances—perhaps something minty in the mid-afternoon and relaxing lavender at bedtime.

And you don't need to go to that extent if it doesn't appeal to you. Everyday aromas such as baking bread, cut flowers, and the fresh scent that follows a rain shower can all initiate good feelings for both of you. If you love Chanel No. 5, take a whiff every now and then or use a scented body lotion that gives you a sensory uplift. If you like the smell, your pleasure hormones will communicate pleasure to your baby. Just steer clear of manufactured scents that contain toxins, including candles and air fresheners. Check the Environmental Working Group website (www.EWG. org) for safe scents.

Taste

Taste is closely connected with smell. Your baby will begin to taste differences in the amniotic fluid at six to seven weeks. Studies have been done to show that babies swallow more frequently when sweet tastes are released into the amniotic fluid and that they swallow less frequently when the mother ingests bitter tastes. This transference happens relatively quickly. It takes forty-five minutes or less for a garlic taste to transfer from mother's ingestion to a perceptible flavor in the amniotic fluid.[25]

Journeywork
Food, Glorious Food

Create a section in your journey book to record what you eat and how the baby physically responds to it about forty-five to sixty minutes later. You can also experiment with communicating the essence of various foods to your baby through your thoughts, voice, and emotions. For example, let's say butterscotch pudding is one of your favorite desserts. Take a spoonful of pudding and savor the sweet, smooth sensation. Describe the taste to your baby and tell them why it's one of your favorites. Stay open to the possibility that your baby may respond with a thought of their own. When you have a sense of what the baby might be communicating, write it down.

This isn't meant to be a record of truth. Instead, it's a speculative dialogue meant to open your mind and heart to receiving messages that your baby may have for you. If you also note any physical responses from the baby forty-five minutes after you eat the pudding, you'll have more clues for your sleuthing.

Be sure to include your favorite healthy foods in this practice. Feeling good about eating fresh, wholesome food can also translate to the baby and may help them to associate positive feelings with nutritional choices.

Sight

Baby can't "see" light outside the womb until about seven months, so for now use your own sense of sight to communicate with your baby by frequently feasting your eyes on beauty. Walking through a park or a flower garden, strolling through an art gallery, and even window shopping can trigger the release of feel-good hormones such as dopamine that produce a sense of well-being for you and the baby. Surround yourself with images that induce feelings of gratitude, awe, peace, and love.

The Sixth Sense

Some of the women we see tell us their pregnancy seems to be enhancing their intuition or sharpening their gut instincts. Since we have four kids of our own, we know firsthand that this can happen. Those intuitive eyes mothers have in the back of their heads are wide open from conception throughout our children's lives.

Many women throughout the world believe that their "sixth sense"—intuition and gut instincts—can foster an eternal bond between mother and baby. This bond transcends time, space, and even death. The unconditional love shared through this bond will strengthen you and give you courage throughout this hero's journey and after the birth of your baby.

We believe this connection is as automatic as the bond formed through the other five senses, even for mothers who are not consciously aware of it. And whether you have frequent intuitive flashes or you've never had a hunch in your life, you can use your sixth sense to facilitate heart-to-heart communication with your baby. In fact, the journeywork and yoga poses in this book were selected with that intention in mind. There's also a practical aspect to this practice. Mothers who have practiced active visualization of positive outcomes for their pregnancy or who have made wishing boards of images that illustrate their vision of healthy, happy children often report easier births, healthier newborns, more positive feelings of belonging between mother and child, and a decreased chance of postpartum depression.

Another bond that's subconscious can be developed in our dream world. When Katie was carrying our first child and dreamed of walking on a beautiful beach while carrying the child in her arms, we wondered if our baby was having the same dream. And if so, was it Katie's dream, the baby's dream, or our dream? These are questions that we probably will not be able to answer with science—at least not in the near future. And this unknown element is another characteristic of your hero's journey. At some point, every mother on this journey leaves the beaten path and strikes out across uncharted territory. There are no words that can adequately capture the depth of each woman's unique experience. You are more alone than you have ever been, and you are more connected than you have ever been. Every thought reflects the duality between the physical and the spiritual. Every heartfelt truth—some running so deep that you can feel them but not find words to speak them—affirms your faith in the mystery of life.

Your dreams, symbolic and literal messages from your subconscious, are worth remembering and capturing in your journey book. Record the events, images, feelings, and messages. If you rarely recall your dreams, write the affirmation "I remember my dreams" and post it where you'll see it several times a day. This intention repeated over time will become believable to your mind and will likely result in your remembering many of your dreams (or at least the most significant parts of them).

To ensure the level of deep sleep that's needed to dream, turn your bedroom into a dreamy sanctuary. Find a way to block out all light. If you need a night light, use one in the red spectrum. Research shows that red light does not disrupt your body's manufacturing of melatonin, the hormone activated by a peaceful, darkened room.[26] And deep, restful sleep is what you need to recharge your body/mind and activate dreaming. The dream state, characterized in sleep studies by rapid eye movements (REM), is partially induced by melatonin.

Keep your journey book or a notepad next to your bed or in the bathroom so you can jot down key words about your dreams to help you remember them. If you dream that you're walking through a field of fragrant flowers with your baby held close to your breast, you might note something like *Flowers/field, baby @ breast*. Even if it seems like a dream has nothing to do with your baby, note it. Dreams are often woven with the fabric of symbolism, so patterns can emerge over time. And if you perceive information about your baby's state of health, as our patient Monica did, tell your ob-gyn. Whether or not your doctor believes in dream communication doesn't matter. What's important is that they hear and respond to your concern with the level of attention or intervention that you and your baby believe is necessary.

Making sure that you're honoring your concerns by getting the attention or intervention that you need is also of prime importance to this stage of your spiritual pregnancy. As your pregnancy progresses, you'll feel more and more attuned to what your baby wants and needs. Some women say they even develop a "knowing" regarding what the growing fetus wants. You may have random thoughts pop into your head or have gut feelings. These are worth your attention and may make more sense if you record them in your journey book so you can see any patterns that may develop.

Learning to trust your instincts and your inner voice will serve you well throughout your pregnancy and beyond. As you move into the second trimester, you will be crossing the first threshold in your hero's journey, and that requires a strong sense of self.

The Spirituality of Pregnancy: From the Ordinary to the Divine

In Jewish tradition, an ordinary act (like eating) can transcend the mundane, becoming divine by surrounding it with blessings and acknowledgments of gratitude to God. There are few things more divine than creating a new life. But the months of pregnancy are also filled with the more immediately tangible but mundane aspects: doctor visits, shopping, balancing work and impending motherhood, and physical discomforts, as well as coping with routine stresses and anxieties—all the "normal" things you had in your life before you became pregnant. But pregnancy, with all its wonders, miracles, and routine processes, is as *kadosh* as it gets.

Kadosh is Hebrew for holy, sanctified, and divine. You are a *k'lei kadosh*—a holy vessel that carries within you the most important of creations: your child. You've engaged in a divine partnership that goes back to the beginning of time—not just with your partner but with God.

Just say the word *kadosh* (kah-doshe) very slowly, letting the word languidly slip from your tongue. Now place your hands on your belly while taking a deep, cleansing breath. Feel the connection you share: you, your baby, your partner, your family (going back through the generations to the beginning of humanity), and God—an embracing, compassionate God—*Eil Rachum*.

Whenever you feel you need centering—or a reminder that what's going on inside your body and in your surroundings is something special—try this simple exercise. With hands on your middle, concentrate on the life within you. (This may be something for your partner to do with you.) You can leave your hands still or massage in a gentle figure-8 effleurage pattern. Breathe in, breath out. "Kadosh." Breathe in, breathe out. "Kadosh."

Like all animals, we humans procreate, duplicating ourselves and ensuring that our legacy continues. But within various cultural and religious traditions, as humans we can elevate the mundane process of pregnancy and childbirth into something separate and special—something holy, spiritual, and divine, or *kadosh*.

To expectant parents, there is nothing ordinary about the birth of a new baby. But pregnancy and childbirth are, in essence, biological processes—natural and ordinary parts of life's cycle. By infusing these wondrous months, full of amazement and new experiences (even if this isn't your first baby), with ritual flavored by tradition, you elevate the journey even higher.

Spiritual Pregnancy Yoga

The spiritual and physical practice of yoga is one of the most supportive habits you can make during your pregnancy. During each trimester there are specific poses that are beneficial for your changing body. Some of these poses help to alleviate physical discomfort, others help to strengthen you for labor and childbirth, and some help you to relax. We recommend that you begin with the following poses and then add the poses offered at the end of part 2 into your practice when you reach your second trimester. When you reach your third trimester, incorporate the poses in part 3 and begin practicing the poses in part 4. If you're accustomed to daily exercise, have practiced yoga before, or are currently practicing yoga, then you can begin doing all of the poses now.

In addition to the physical benefits, yoga is a gateway to higher awareness. The most important aspect of practicing prenatal yoga is one that is practiced in all yoga, which is *ahimsa,* or nonviolence to yourself and others. This means paying attention to your body and only doing poses that feel good. As your baby grows and changes positions, certain poses may not feel good to you, even if they've felt great before. Never force yourself into a position because you have been able to do it in the past. This is inappropriate and can cause strain or injury. Always get permission from your doctor or healthcare provider prior to beginning any prenatal exercise.

. . . .

The yoga poses and photos throughout the book are provided by Jennifer (Wolfe) More, creator of Vinyasa Prenatal Yoga and founder of Dolphin Yoga and Doula Training.

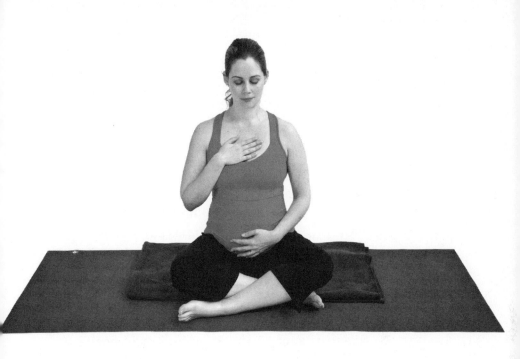

Yoga Pose
. . . .
Seated Hand on Heart
Integrating Two Lives

This yoga pose releases you from all outside thoughts and concerns and allows you to deeply connect with your baby by melding your life forces and strengthening your spiritual union.

Sit on a yoga pillow or a blanket folded into a firm square.

Place one hand on your heart and the other on your belly. (It doesn't matter which hand. Try it with your right hand on your belly and then your left, and see what feels most comfortable to you.)

Take two or three full, deep breaths.

Mentally scan your body to increase your awareness of how you are feeling in this moment.

Continue breathing deeply and slowly, allowing your lungs to fill up completely before gently exhaling. If you feel lightheaded or have any discomfort, shift your position or lie down.

Imagine a golden-orange glow in your womb. Imagine you can feel the warmth of this glow in the palm of your hand.

Now, imagine you can see a vibrant green light glowing in your heart. Feel the vitality of this energy radiating against in the palm of your hand.

Visualize the orange light in your womb expanding to encompass your entire body.

Now, visualize the green light in your heart expanding to encompass your entire body. With each inhalation, see the green light filling your body with unconditional love. With each exhalation, see the orange light filling your body with a powerful life force.

Continue to alternate colors with inhaling (green) and exhaling (orange) for one or two minutes.

Open your mouth and say "ahhhhh" as the breath of life flows freely from your lungs, taking with it any anxiety or distress that you may have been feeling.

Focus on the unconditional love and life force of these energy centers as they merge with one another. Imagine that you can see and feel the combined energy of life and love enveloping your baby. Smile as your heart and your womb radiate the powerful light that you and the baby are creating together.

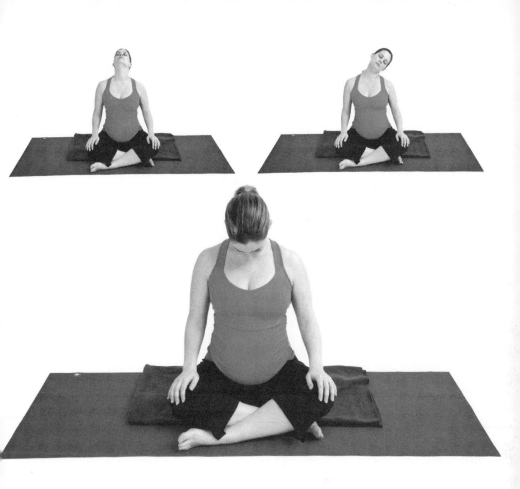

Yoga Pose
Seated Head Rolls
Releasing the Mind

Relaxing your neck and keeping your spine long, roll
your head a few times slowly to the right, then a few
times slowly to the left. This pose releases tension in the
head, neck, and shoulders. It also releases thoughts and
thought processes that can keep you from being present
and living in the moment.

Benefits

- Practicing seated hand-on-heart and head rolls are nice ways to begin a stretching routine or prenatal class. These yoga poses will help you to tune in to your body before you begin moving.

- Use these poses to ground and center yourself in a place of quiet mindfulness. Being present with your body and with baby in the moment will guide you in moving and stretching.

Precautions

- Every day in pregnancy is different, so let your body be your guide with regard to the yoga poses you practice.

- Be gentle with yourself, and remember that it's good to rest when you need it.

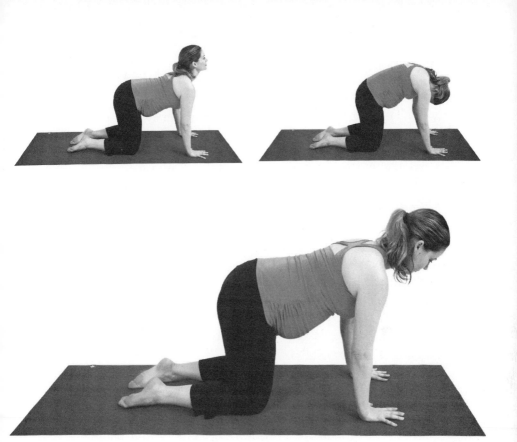

Yoga Pose
Cat/Cow
Grounding

To move into Cat/Cow, begin on your hands and knees. Make sure your hands are directly under your shoulders.

On the inhalation, straighten your spine, lift your head, and gaze as though seeing from a point between your eyebrows. (This is "Cow.")

On the exhalation, press your hands into your yoga mat and round your back, tucking your tailbone under. (This is "Cat.")

Exaggerate the roundness of your back by pressing your hands into the mat.

This is a pose that should be done every day.

Benefits

- If the baby is in an uncomfortable position,
  the rocking of the pelvis will help them
  to turn and get comfortable.

- Releases back tension

- Increases spine flexibility and strength

- During labor, this position can help to turn the
  baby into a position that is more comfortable
  for you and more conducive for birthing.

Precautions

- Be sure not to sway your back too much, especially
  in the third trimester, because this can put too much
  strain on your spine from the weight of your baby.

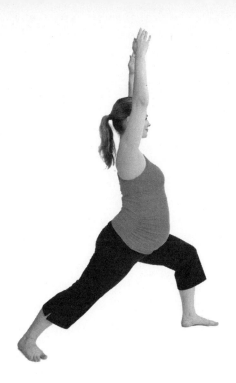

Yoga Pose
Warrior I
Stamina, Balance, and Strength

From a standing position where your feet are hip-width apart, step one foot back about 3½ to 4 feet. Keep the back foot at a 45-degree angle as you bring your arms above your head and dip slowly down into the pose. It is important to only go as low as is comfortable for you.
   Hold for 1 to 3 breaths.

Benefits
  • Improves balance
  • Increases strength

Precautions
As your pregnancy progresses, be sure you are centered and grounded. If you feel unsteady, you can hold onto

a chair or place one hand against a wall. However, if you think you may still lose your balance, skip this pose.

Approaching the First Threshold

During the past few months you've discovered aspects of yourself that you didn't know existed. You've tuned in to the voice of inner guidance, and you've reached out for the support that you desire and require for the path ahead. Brava! Give yourself a big pat on the back, and give your growing baby belly a soft pat too. You and your baby have been traveling together for a quarter of a year now, and with each day you'll get to know each other a little better. As you leave the first trimester behind and cross the first threshold on your hero's journey, you are physically and symbolically surrendering to the world of motherhood and all that it entails.

Part 2
Second Trimester

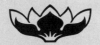

Crossing the First Threshold

As your pregnancy moves into the second trimester, you'll find yourself entering what many women call the honeymoon phase of pregnancy. This is your "You look fabulous, darling" phase. Hormones rushing through your system add luster to your hair and skin. You begin showing, but people will still hesitate before assuming you're pregnant. You may still be able to fit into your pre-pregnancy clothes, but not for long. Soon your belly will begin to protrude, and you'll become more physically aware of the life growing inside you. Morning sickness is letting up, bacon smells good again, and you begin to feel a renewed sense of energy and well-being.

Now is the time to stand in your strength as a mother-to-be and enjoy the moment. It's also the time to have passionate and climactic sex and deepen your bond with your partner. Many women rave about second trimester sex, and with your inner and outer glow, you'll be more gloriously sexy than ever. Plus, love-making can reduce your anxiety and stress and create a warm love vibe for the baby. Unless you're having a high-risk pregnancy, sex shouldn't cause any problems for the baby. Some physicians even say it's good for the baby to be moved around and massaged by the physical movements and vibrations.

As a spiritually aware mother-to-be, we encourage you to revel in this midplace in the journey. During this magical time, the life growing inside you takes shape, heft, and substance, and this life force shines through you, creating that beautiful mother-to-be radiance.

Second Trimester:
What's Happening?

Month Four

Physically

- The baby is floating freely in the amniotic fluid of your womb.

- Now the baby can suck a thumb, clasp hands, flex arms, and kick legs.

- During this month, the baby doubles in length and triples in weight, measuring 3 to 5 inches long and weighing about 2 ounces.

Spiritually

As the baby floats freely in your womb, you may find the sensations calming and soothing. There are many spiritual practices that involve sacred water, and for the baby, your amniotic fluid is as sacred as life itself. Many women say they frequently have "happy tears" this month as they appreciate and marvel at their body's ability to hold, protect, and nurture new life. Take a few minutes each day to place your hands on your growing belly, close your eyes, breathe deeply, and imagine that you and your baby are floating together in a warm and beautiful pool of crystal-clear water. Communicate your love and be receptive to receiving love.

Month Five
Physically

- Baby's ears are developing, and so is their hearing. Soon, they will be able to hear your voice, music, and other external sounds.

- Baby's legs are about as big as your little finger, and you are starting to feel flutters of them kicking.

- By the end of the month, your baby is 8 to 10 inches long and weighs about a half pound.

Spiritually

As baby's sense of hearing develops, a new gateway for sharing your love opens. Even if you never sing, not even in the shower, you may feel called to sing to your baby. Songs like "Twinkle Twinkle Little Star" that you'd all but forgotten may spring to mind and surprise you. Go with it. No matter what opinion you have of your singing voice, baby is certain to love it. Now is also a great time to introduce your baby to beautiful, harmonious music. Notice whether the baby responds to a particular song or rhythm. Some mothers say that the songs that put their baby to sleep in the womb are the same songs that lull them to sleep after birth.

Month Six

Physically

- Baby's eyelids, eyelashes, and eyebrows are now developed.

- Full-fledged kicking is now strong enough that you and your partner can both feel it.

- Air sacs are beginning to form in the baby's lungs.

- By the end of this trimester, your baby is about a foot long and weighs about one pound.

Spiritually

Physical life begins with the first breath and ends with the last, but spiritual life is thought to be eternal. During this month, as baby's lungs are developing, you may start to feel short of breath. Now that baby is getting bigger and taking up more space, your lungs may sometimes feel constricted. As you adjust your position, practice taking deep, full breaths, breathing in not just oxygen but the universal energy, or prana, you need to be strong, healthy, and centered during this time.

Chapter 3

Initiation to Motherhood

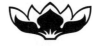

Your legs will get heavy and tired.
Then comes a moment of feeling
the wings you've grown, lifting.
Rumi

Rachel sniffed as she pulled another tissue from her pocket. "I never used to cry, and now I'm crying all the time, when I'm sad *and* when I'm happy. Is this a hormone thing?"

Many women entering the second trimester of their journey feel more emotionally tender or even raw. This "uber-sensitive" time is perfect for opening wider and deeper to your spirit and the spirit of your child. Allowing yourself to feel the depths of your emotions while at the same time seeking inner peace through quiet time, meditation, and yoga is an important part of your hero's journey. Like Rachel, your heightened emotional sensitivity is being caused by hormonal and physical changes—but that's not all. The increasing reality that *you* are the divine vessel for a new life tends to spark and intensify your sensitivity for life itself.

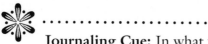

Journaling Cue: In what ways do you feel your body and spirit bonding to your baby's today?

During your first trimester, your baby was in a relatively form-less state of pure potential. As the baby grows and you become more aware of their presence, you may find yourself feeling a little anxious. Sometimes, the transition from pure potential to physical reality is a frightening one. This is going to be a real child who will experience joy and sorrow, pain and pleasure, success and fail-ure. In your hero's journey, this shift to the solid realities of life is the bridge between departure and initiation. During your first trimester, in a real sense you departed on your journey, leaving the ordinary world behind. Now you are engaged in the initiation stage of the hero's journey, where you will encounter new chal-lenges, make new allies, and begin to learn the rules of this new world.

And the baby is changing right along with you. They are grow-ing (and may weigh as much as two pounds by now), sprout-ing hair, growing fingernails, and beginning to suck tiny thumbs. Ears are forming, and they can now hear your heart beating, your voice, and other sounds outside your womb. And by week fifteen or sixteen, an ultrasound can show whether you're carrying a boy or a girl. Whether you choose to find out the gender of your baby or not, it's fun to be aware that the question has been decided.

Scientists have also done studies on whether or not prenatal ultrasounds changed the way babies bond with parents before birth. One study discovered that the father/baby connection was boosted after an ultrasound, although mother/baby bonding was unchanged.[27] The study's scientists believed that the reason moms' scores for emotional bonding didn't go up after seeing their baby in an ultrasound was because in most cases, the internal dynamics of becoming a mother were bonding her to the baby in ever deepening ways. It was unnecessary for moms to see visual proof of that bonding, as they felt it in their bodies every day.

The Quickening

"For me, one of the most thrilling moments is feeling my baby move for the first time," said Heather as she gently pushed her hands into her blossoming belly. Heather had been a patient of ours for years, and the baby she was carrying was her third. But no matter how many times you've been pregnant, that first sensation of movement, called the quickening, is a miracle moment. "Time stops, and everything around me disappears. For that moment, me and my baby are the only two people on the planet," Heather said with a smile.

You can look forward to this miracle moment around week eighteen or nineteen, when you'll feel a fluttering sensation when baby moves in your womb. If this isn't your first pregnancy, you have more relaxed and sensitive uterus muscles and might feel these flutters as early as week fourteen or fifteen. In terms of your epic journey, this is the time in legends and lore when divine or supernatural helpers come to aid the hero after a series of tests or trials. In world myth and shared culture, this phase of the hero's journey corresponds to the finding of the Holy Grail, to Psyche realizing the unseen lover is her true beloved, or even to Cinderella getting help from her fairy godmother to dress up and go to the ball. By superimposing the template of the three trimesters on your journey, this middle trimester is characterized by the blissful experience of connecting with the divine in yourself, your child, and the world at large. Experiencing the physical reality of your child is akin to the hero discovering the ultimate boon. Symbolically, the Holy Grail—the sacred chalice—is the developing physical body of your baby.

In Hindu tradition, rituals are held before the child is born to facilitate healthy transition from the world of spirit to the world of flesh. In the ritual called Valaikappu, the adorning with bangles, the mother of the mother-to-be places twenty bangles in her daughter's left hand and twenty-one bangles in her right hand. The bangles represent various forms of protection and prayers for mother and baby, and they are not removed until the mother goes into labor. In Catholic tradition, the second trimester is beautifully illustrated with the story of the Visitation, in which Elizabeth conceived John the Baptist when she was in her forties and believed her advanced years would prevent her from becoming pregnant. When Mary, Elizabeth's younger cousin, greeted Elizabeth, John leaped in her womb and "Elizabeth herself was filled with the Holy Spirit so that she cried out with a loud voice, 'Blessed art thou among women, and blessed is the fruit of thy womb.'"[28] As the weight of your child increases and you become more aware of their movements, baby's awareness of your movements will be increasing too. When they respond to your touch or the soft coo and murmur of your voice, you too may feel "visited" by the divine force of life that embodies both baby and you.

Journeywork
Focusing Breath Meditation

Sometimes called the counting breath, this is a technique used in Zen practice.

Sit in a comfortable position with your spine straight and your head inclined slightly forward.

Gently close your eyes, take a few deep breaths, then let the breath come naturally without trying to influence it. Ideally it will be quiet and slow, but depth and rhythm may vary.

To begin the exercise, silently count *one* as you exhale. The next time you exhale, count up to two as you exhale. On the third exhale, count up to three as you exhale, and so on, up to five. Then begin a new cycle, counting *one* on the next exhalation.

Don't intentionally count higher than five, and count only as you exhale. You will know your attention has wandered when you find yourself up to eight, twelve, or even nineteen!

Try to do ten minutes of this form of meditation daily.

Favorable Practices

As flesh, blood, and bone develop within you, your relationship with baby and baby's relationship with you expands and deepens. This is a time when you'll probably spend a lot of time thinking about what's best for baby and you. As you become more aware of how your choices affect baby, every decision feels big. *How much sleep should I be getting? Is it really okay to have one glass of red wine a couple times a week? When I'm stressed out, can baby feel that?* In general, the rule of thumb is that if it's good for you, it's good for baby, but remember that this does not apply to drugs and alcohol, and baby will want a much smaller amount than you, so use discretion and moderation.

Up until the 1990s when we learned that smoke was bad for developing babies, it wasn't uncommon for women to smoke when they were pregnant. Babies were exposed to secondhand smoke because we didn't know it could harm them. Shawn has seen photos of his mother breastfeeding him in the late 1960s with three of her friends, and all four of them are smoking in the house with him latched to the breast. It's no wonder he had chronic ear infections as a child. Since people thought the quality of the environment the baby was in was not a concern, the idea that the environment *inside* the womb could affect a baby would have been written off as superstition or just plain malarkey.

But we now know that baby can benefit from your exercise, nutrition, and clean conditions, and we can also see how a mother's choices can negatively affect a pregnancy. In our current state of chronic stress, fatigue, and technology overload, it is important to buffer yourself from these influences by occasionally detoxing from the stimulus. You can calm baby by simply breathing deeply or listening to comforting music.

Journeywork
Yogic Breathing

To get energized or calm down at any time of day or night, practice the following breathing exercises. They will also cleanse and nourish you and the baby with the energy of prana, or breath power. Reproduced with permission from Andrew Weil, these exercises also demonstrate how breathing can be both stimulating and meditative when done different ways.

**The Stimulating Breath
(also called the Bellows Breath)**
The Stimulating Breath is adapted from a yogic breathing technique. Use this breathing exercise to raise your vital energy and increase alertness. Try it the next time you need an energy boost.

Inhale and exhale rapidly through your nose, keeping your mouth closed but relaxed. Your breaths in and out should be equal in duration, but as short as possible. This is a noisy breathing exercise.

Try for three in-and-out breath cycles per second. This produces a quick movement of the diaphragm, suggesting a bellows. Breathe normally after each cycle.

Do not do for more than fifteen seconds on your first try. Each time you practice the Stimulating Breath, you can increase your time by five seconds or so, until you reach a full minute.

If done properly, you may feel invigorated, comparable to the heightened awareness you feel after a good workout. You should feel the effort in the back of your neck and diaphragm, chest, and abdomen.

The 4-7-8 Relaxing Breath
This exercise is a natural tranquilizer for the nervous system. Unlike tranquilizing drugs, which often lose their power over time, this exercise will work forever. The effects are subtle when you first try it but become stronger with repetition and practice. This exercise is simple, takes almost no time, requires no equipment, and can be done anywhere. Although you can do the exercise in any position, sit with your back straight while learning it.

Place the tip of your tongue against the ridge of tissue just behind your upper front teeth and keep it there throughout the exercise. You will be exhaling through your mouth around your tongue. Try pursing your lips slightly if this feels awkward.

Exhale completely through your mouth, making a whoosh sound.

Close your mouth and inhale quietly through your nose as you mentally count to four.

Hold your breath for a silent count of seven.

Exhale completely through your mouth, making a whoosh sound to a count as you mentally count to eight.

This completes one breath. Repeat the cycle three times for a total of four breaths, breathing normally between breaths. We recommend doing this at least twice a day. You cannot do it too frequently. Keep in mind that you always inhale quietly through your nose and exhale audibly through your mouth, and that exhalation takes twice as long as inhalation. The time you spend on each breath is not important; the ratio of 4:7:8 is important. If you have trouble holding your breath, speed the exercise up but keep to the ratio of 4:7:8. With practice you can slow it all down and get used to inhaling and exhaling more deeply.

Do not do more than four breaths at one time for the first month of practice. Later, if you wish, you can extend it to eight breaths. If you feel a little lightheaded when you first breathe this way, sit down, and don't be concerned; it will pass.

Once you develop this technique by practicing it every day, it will be a very useful tool that you will always have. Use it whenever anything upsetting happens—*before* you react. Use it whenever you're feeling stressed and to help you fall asleep. This breathing exercise is highly encouraged. Everyone can benefit from it.

Journeywork
. . . .
Releasing Fear

It's not unusual for worries to try to hijack your peace of mind: *Will my baby be healthy? Will the birth be difficult? What if there are complications?* These anxieties are all characteristic of the initiation stage of your epic journey. Use them as incentive to train yourself to elicit inner peace, joy, and trust—in yourself and in the spiritual universe. And use them to practice listening to your intuition and paying attention to your gut instincts.

Take out your journey book. For the next five minutes, write down the questions or worries that are weighing heavily on you. Get in touch with what's at the root of each worry, concern, or question. Why are you worried? Why is this question so important? What has sparked this anxiety? Writing your fears is like shining a light on them. It freezes these mental demons in their tracks and allows you to capture their essence. Once you have them pinned to the page, you can deal with them one by one.

Once you've completed your answers, let them sit for a day or so. Then come back to them and circle the ones that still have power over you. These are the ones to discuss with your doctor, doula, or spiritual pregnancy mentors.

Sorting out the mental clutter will help you make good decisions about the practices to embrace until your child is born. This is an important part of the journey that all pregnant women walk, and it has given rise to many world customs and beliefs about how the mother-to-be should conduct herself.

For example, Jewish mystics instructed new mothers to wait until the midpoint in their pregnancy to reveal the news that they were with child, believing that the soul enters the infant's body when the mother's belly is obviously brimming with life. Some traditions believe that you should avoid people and events that evoke anger, anxiety, fear, and other emotions that are upsetting to you; we think this is a very favorable practice throughout life, but particularly during your spiritual pregnancy. There is considerable science and plenty of personal and clinical experience to convince us that chemicals your emotions produce affect your developing baby. And there's no longer any dispute that what you eat, drink, and breathe has a direct effect on your developing baby.

Long before modern medicine discovered that the child was partaking of whatever the mother ate, drank, or smoked, some cultures, including the people of the Six Nations, enforced the practice of pregnant women abstaining from smoke and alcohol. They were not allowed to use these substances lest their children come into the world intoxicated. Women with child were also not permitted to receive or hear bad news or walk in unclean places or near bodies or burials. The delicate spiritual state of the unborn and the thin barrier between the child and the spirit world meant that pregnant women should guard their thoughts and actions at all times to ensure positive, strength-affirming energy flowed into and around the unborn baby. Aboriginal culture, as well as some African groups like the San people in the Kalahari, have similar spiritual traditions.

Journeywork
A Bad News "Fast"

Take a page from the hallowed traditions of ancient cultures and do a bad news "fast": for 24 to 48 hours, avoid seeing, hearing, or talking about bad news or feelings. When a worry or negative thought crosses your mind, silently repeat a mantra like "My child is growing perfectly healthy inside me" or "My baby will be whole, healthy, and strong." Write a few mantras that resonate with you and keep them on hand until you've memorized them. Skip the newspaper and news shows, and resist the temptation to surf the Internet. Watch movies that are inspiring or funny and avoid the chillers, thrillers, and sad endings. If your favorite TV shows have disturbing images or stressful elements, avoid them too. Let the world turn without you for a few days, and you'll feel refreshed, infused with positive vibes, and more focused on baby's movements and inner direction. We recommend doing frequent bad news fasts. Take out your day planner and schedule a couple of these each month for the remainder of your pregnancy.

Pregnant women in Irish culture embraced the ancient belief that in mid-pregnancy the fetus is living partly in the spirit world and is vulnerable to thoughts and wishes from that world as well as the world of the living. Women were encouraged to have positive and affirming thoughts and to speak lovingly to the new life inside them. Since Irish culture honors the power of words and names, this is also traditionally a time when the new mother considers the right name for her child and may also name the child's godparents, the guardians of the baby's spiritual upbringing. And as singing can be just as important to the Irish as talking, the tradition of singing to the unborn was and still is an important part of Irish tradition. Fathers in particular were encouraged to sing to their unborn children so that the babies would know them when they were born.

Up until the 1930s, many doctors advised women to refrain from swimming, and in 1921, the book *Hygiene de la maman et de bebe (Hygiene of the Mother and Child)* by Leon Pouliot cautioned women against riding on streetcars, walking through shops, and reorganizing their kitchen cupboards. Other doctors said pregnant women should not use sewing machines or ride horses or bikes. So, like today, women were getting a lot of confusing information. And, like today, women were listening to their intuition and perhaps their spirit guides in choosing their own favorable practices. Many women in the nineteenth and early twentieth centuries wore religious ribbons or medals to protect their developing babies and help ward off evil. For as long as woman have been giving birth, this awe-inspiring event has motivated ritualistic offerings and prayers to gods, goddesses, angels, saints, and ancestors.

And it's also inspired myths. We're not sure where or why cats got such a bad rap, but we've heard the old wives' tales that say a cat can steal a baby's spirit and that a cat can take away a baby's breath. We've also heard modern-day myths that say pregnant women should not share company with cats, and this sadly leads to countless feline friends being dropped off at animal shelters every year. For the record, the only aspect of having a cat that can be harmful to you is their feces. You have to ingest and/or inhale them to get the disease called *Toxoplasma gondii (T. gondii)*, so as long as you wear gloves when you clean the litter box and thoroughly wash your hands after removing the gloves, there won't be a problem. Of course, this could also be a great time to turn the litter box cleaning over to your partner or teach your older kids to take on this responsibility. (For more details, visit the National Humane Society website).[29]

Some Jewish mothers-to-be in mystical traditions use a prayer or a saying from the Torah as a meditative tool that helps keep them focused on the spiritual growth of the baby and the connection they share. The mantra is a gentle reminder to bring straying thoughts back to the center of our soul. These types of prayer rituals can awaken us to spiritual truths. The daily practice of being mindful of our external and internal world helps us to stay centered and spiritually connected.

With the second trimester well underway, you've devoted time and consideration to deciding which favorable practices you want to adopt for the remainder of your pregnancy and which practices you want to avoid. You've probably felt the baby's early stirrings inside your womb (or you soon will), and this dramatically increases the reality that you're becoming a mother. While you may have been making an effort to be healthy all along, many women feel a surge in their desire to eat right, exercise, and destress with yoga after the quickening. And as your body visibly changes with each passing week, you will feel more and more like the mother that you are becoming.

Chapter 4

Entering the Stage of Bliss

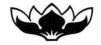

*May every living thing
be full of bliss.*
The Dhammapada

"I love imagining what he looks like and if he'll look like his dad," said our patient, whom we'll call Monica, as she stepped onto the scale during her checkup. "Sometimes I close my eyes and pretend I can see his face, and then I fast-forward and imagine I can see him when he's born and at his first birthday party or his first day of school. I wonder if he'll play the guitar like his dad or play soccer like me or both or neither," she said with a little laugh.

As you approach the midpoint of this spiritual journey, you will find your thoughts are increasingly preoccupied with being a mom and wondering what your new baby will be like. Why not ask your baby? Invite them to join your daydreams or visualizations. Some women are surprised when thoughts seem to pop into their heads that they'd never had before and feel certain these are thoughts from the baby or the baby's spirit. Our friend Karen said:

Just about everyone in our family is artistic, so I kept wondering if my baby would paint, sketch, do pottery, make jewelry, or be a photographer. One day, when I was thinking about this, I asked out loud, "What sort of artist are you, baby?" At that moment, an image like you'd see on the cover of *Bon Appetit* popped into my head. "A culinary artist? A chef?" I asked out loud. I couldn't believe it when baby gave me three swift kicks.

We love Karen's story, but even if her baby hadn't physically responded, we would have suggested she describe the experience she had and the image she saw in her journey book. Just like learning to serve a tennis ball takes practice and repetition, so does learning this new form of communication with your baby. Practice not with the goal to get the "right answers" but with the intention to explore the unknown together.

Every day offers new opportunities for discovery and bonding, and this can be done in very simple ways. When you're choosing between an orange and a pear, ask the baby if they have a preference and go with whatever pops into your mind or any physical reaction that the baby provides. Resist the urge to overthink this. A common question we get is, "What if he kicks when I say pear? Does that mean he wants one or he doesn't?" Honestly, at this stage, it doesn't really matter. This is a great way to learn together over time. Just pick one and notice how you feel for the next half hour or so. If you feel good, you made a good choice for you and baby regardless of their preference. If you feel bad, choose something different next time. You can also experiment by offering baby just one choice at a time. Try picking up some different fruits or vegetables and asking baby about each one.

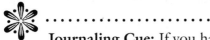

Journaling Cue: If you have a sense that any of your food choices are getting a positive or negative reaction, note it in your journey book for future investigation.

Some mothers-to-be find that imagining their babies growing and developing helps them to bond. At this stage your baby is enveloped in a coating of fine hair (lanugo) that helps keep them warm until body fat develops. The baby has eyelashes and eyebrows and may be able to sense some light outside the womb. By the end of this trimester, your baby will be about twelve inches long and may weigh as much as a pound. This is also the period where the organs and systems are growing and maturing. Just as you are walking with a foot in the spiritual and the physical worlds, so is your baby. They are journeying toward the twenty-four-week mark, when a fetus is considered a viable human being.

Communicating with Sound and Music

At about week nineteen, your baby's tiny, shell-like ears will be able to hear sounds from their inner and outer worlds. That means your baby can hear your voice! And they may be able to hear Dad's voice even better because lower frequencies penetrate the abdomen and amniotic fluids easier than high frequencies. This is a great way for Dad to bond with baby too. And when the two of you are enjoying talking to each other, we think that the baby can sense that too. Keep in mind that the baby's soundscape doesn't just include Mommy and Daddy's voices. It also includes the sound of your heartbeat, the rhythm of your breath, and your sighs, coughs, and digestive processes all through the soft, muffling barrier of amniotic fluid. Perhaps this distant memory of half-muffled talk is the reason why the sound of voices in other rooms is so hypnotically intriguing to us—it reminds us of the time when the entire world sounded this way from within our mother's womb.

During this trimester and the next, experiment with different types of music and notice how the baby responds. Sink into your body/mind and let your intuition interpret the baby's movements. Does the baby find this music calming or invigorating?

It has been suggested that developing babies respond to different types of music and can even differentiate different composers. It may be the composer's use of minor or major keys or the increased use of deep bass and drums during symphonies. For those women who like rock or louder types of music, keep in mind that the baby definitely could be stimulated by the sounds. If you're not soothed by the music, then chances are neither is your baby. It's okay to play loud rock music sometimes, but play some more soothing music as well. Remember that, like you, the baby is developing a discerning taste for tunes, and exposing them to different types of music is a fun way to share what you love.

Journeywork
Musical Moves

Baby has developing tastes and loves to hear different sounds. Studies have shown babies move with the cadence of your unique voice, and they also move in different patterns to various kinds of music. Sit down with your journey book and a pen, along with an MP3 player or next to a stereo speaker. Play the music at a level loud enough for your baby to hear, but not too loud. Introduce baby to a variety of music, including classical, country, rock, easy listening, New Age, and Big Band. As you listen to the music together, record fetal kicks and note how the baby moves.

Does the baby move vigorously or with such force that it almost hurts or is there a smooth gentleness to the movements, as if the baby is doing a water dance in your belly?

Journaling Cue: Record the findings and reflect on how you felt during the song as well. Chances are there is some correlation between your response to the music and the baby's response.

Mothers-to-be have long believed that music, singing, and talking to the baby is a good thing, even though science has just recently been substantiating that inner wisdom. Psychological researchers Anthony DeCasper and Melanie Spence have conducted studies revealing that babies who were repeatedly read the same books in utero recognized those books after birth and were comforted with the same readings. This obviously points to the idea that babies in utero recognize and remember certain sounds. Pre-birth communication is intriguing and just beginning to be understood on a medical and scientific level.

It's important at this stage in your journey to understand that your baby's awareness of the world is ever-widening. Your own journey as a mother is now moving inward to meet your new child. As the physical contours of baby's body take shape, you can spiritually acclimate yourself to the vital and separate person you will bring into the world. Some mothers-to-be use the second trimester to work on pre-birth communication. Others journal or write letters to their babies, knowing that one day they will pass down these messages from pre-birth time when their child is old enough to understand them. The important dynamic to work with here is the movement from *becoming* to *being*.

Finding Your Still Center

With the second trimester being so physically and spiritually trans-formative, it's not surprising that so many of our patients experience a little more stress and chaos than they'd like. First-time mothers-to-be tend to feel a little more stressed out during this time than those who are pregnant for the second or third time. But women who already have children tend to have more chaos to deal with in juggling the needs of their unborn child, their own needs, and the needs of their children, not to mention work and other daily demands.

As the miraculous process of becoming takes place inside you, it's even more important to keep a still center. So much is happening and is about to happen, but you can take wisdom from many world cultures and use this time to draw inward and create an open, still center point that will ground you through the changes to come.

Have you ever seen a whirling dervish? This sect of the Islamic mystic Sufi order practices a moving meditation designed to bring the participant closer to the Beloved, or God. These famous practitioners spin like tops wearing long, flowing white robes and tall hats. Their skirts are designed to move around their bodies like transfixing waves. The movement is done to the sound of drums and a flute. If you ever see it, you'll never forget it, just because it's amazing to watch. But if you look closer, you'll learn a secret.

Beneath that whirling top of a skirt, the dervish keeps one foot solidly in place. It moves on that place but never strays from that spot. Beneath the top hat, the head is tilted. This keeps the dervish's inner ear fluid stable so he won't get dizzy. And the flower-like motion of his upheld arm is a focal point. If the dervish opens his eyes at all, he looks at the focal point and regains equilibrium like a ballerina does by "spotting" a corner of a room during pirouettes. This is a physical example of connecting to and being grounded by a still point.

During your second trimester, you might find yourself physically and emotionally experiencing a dizzying sensation. This can be caused by rising hormones and by the growing pressure of your uterus on the large vein called the vena cava, which carries deoxygenated blood from the lower half of your body back to your heart. Your uterus also pushes on the sciatic and femoral nerves.

Mentally and emotionally, the dizzying sensation can be triggered when you're stressed out or overwhelmed. Centering yourself like the dervish and finding your still point of oneness is a way to move inward during this stage of your journey. The theory of *wahdat al-wujûd*, or unity of being, is part of Sufi metaphysics. Rumi, the great Sufi poet and philosopher, concentrated much of his work on speaking about achieving this unity through connection with the Godforce as Beloved. When you still the outer world and listen for the voice of your beloved, you achieve oneness with God. Rumi says:

> Make everything in you an ear, each atom of your being, and you will hear at every moment what the Source is whispering to you, just to you and for you, without any need for my words or anyone else's. You are—we all are—the beloved of the Beloved, and in every moment, in every

event of your life, the Beloved is whispering to you exactly what you need to hear and know. Who can ever explain this miracle? It simply is. Listen, and you will discover it every passing moment. Listen, and your whole life will become a conversation in thought and act between you and Him, directly, wordlessly, now and always.[30]

Some Sufi traditions also have a meditation practice that corresponds with this thought, called the Heart Meditation, or Meditation on the Beloved. In this practice you reserve time every day to meditate on the object of your love and on the feeling of love inside you. The Sufis believe that the emotion of love in the heart is stronger than wandering thoughts in the mind and that by going directly to the path of the beloved, you invoke the power of the heart—seen by some Sufi artists as a heart with wings—to move you to oneness with the creator.

Journeywork
Heart-Centering Meditation

Set aside time on three consecutive days to do this meditation. Three is a mystical number, and it represents permanence and adds strength to our acts. Once you do this meditation three days in a row, you may decide you want to do it every day.

Sit comfortably in a chair or on cushions on the floor (if you can get up without getting dizzy). Begin with a few minutes of yogic breathing from chapter 3.

When you feel your breath calming you to the point of receptiveness, move your awareness to the child within you. Send your baby waves of love. Imagine warm blankets of love wrapping your baby in comfort and joy. Imagining baby snuggling closer and gurgling for joy as he or she opens, relaxes, and receives this heart-centered gift of love. Now take a few minutes to breathe.

Reverse the meditation and imagine baby sending you waves of love, comfort, and joy. Imagine your body glowing from the love radiating from your womb. See the umbilical cord that binds you to the baby as a golden cord feeding love back and forth between you and your child. Now take a few more yogic pranayama breaths. Center yourself again. Radiate the love from you and your child outward toward the world, to the street where you live, to the people you know.

Now move that love further and extend it to those you don't know—the people in your country, your continent. Now move that love even further out and extend it to all living creatures in the world: the four-legged, finned, and feathered ones. Take one more deep breath. Now move that love beyond our world to the entire universe.

Next, draw in more pranic energy through five deep breaths and move that powerful love back to the creator, to God as you know him or her. Imagine you and the Godforce connected by a golden umbilical cord the way you and your baby are connected. Now imagine God sending you warm waves of love, infusing and enveloping you and the baby in a golden globe of light.

Variations of this meditation are used in many spiritual traditions, although it is particularly popular in Buddhist thought and mystic traditions like Sufism. Christians can use Christ-centered imagery for this powerful centering technique. New mothers from Jewish traditions may wish to use the image or sound of the name of God, which is always written without one of its vowels to accord the Creator the mystery of the holy name.

Pair this exercise with yogic breathing for a more powerful grounding experience. You may also wish to practice gentle yogic movement before or after the meditation.

Warming Your Love Connection

"I never dreamed that the best sex I've ever had would be now, while I'm pregnant," Michelle said, laughing. "I hear ya, lady," said Karla, another woman in our focus group. Pretty soon, all the new moms-to-be were chiming in about their new lease on lovemaking as the "veterans" smiled knowingly.

During the second trimester of your pregnancy, your body is primed to enjoy some of the hottest, most satisfying sex that you'll ever have. The hormones that your body is producing to make sure the baby develops properly can produce an aphrodisiac effect. We can't say that all women in the middle stage of their pregnancies enjoy this side effect, but there's a good chance that you'll notice a lift in your libido. But whether you feel more passionate or not, this can be a wonderful time along your journey to strengthen your spiritual and physical bond with your partner. There is no doubt that being new parents or adding another child to your family adds a little more work, and—at least for a while—a little less play. Sexually and spiritually bonding with each other at this time is a wise investment in your marriage. And these magical moments that you share will also go a long way toward making the sexless time after birthing more tolerable for both of you.

Some couples find that this is the perfect time for them to explore tantric sex. This practice, which emerged in India more than 6,000 years ago, is a pathway to reclaiming the sexual intimacy that many believe is our birthright. The ancient art of Tantra is designed to open our hearts, allow us to experience our emotions more fully, and express our divine love through sexuality. The practice of Tantra originated as a rebellious response to organized religion that put forth the idea that people should abstain from sexual practices if they wanted to reach enlightenment. Tantra defied these ascetic beliefs by asserting that sex could be a gateway to the Divine and that all earthly pleasures were sacred acts when done with the intention to honor and connect with the Divine.

Whether or not you explore Tantra, the skin-to-skin, heart-to-heart time you spend with your partner is a win-win for both of you—and, we believe, for baby too. When we share this with our patients, some women actually wince. This is so sad! But, because of Western culture's stereotypes of tiny-waisted women being sexy, you may not like the way you look naked right now. We're inviting you to suspend that cultural perspective and view your blossoming belly, full breasts, and widening hips as the manifestation of the gorgeously sacred transformation that's occurring.

Journeywork
Falling in Love with
Your Goddess Self

Remove your clothing and stand in front of a full-length mirror. Slowly turn around and look at your body as a silent, objective observer. Pretend you have never seen a human body, so you have no judgments about what looks pleasing and what doesn't. Take an objective assessment from an out-of-body point of view: "This female has fair skin with freckles and reddish-brown hair. Her eyes are green. Her breasts are the size of grapefruits and look like they would bounce easily. Her belly is rounding like the bottom of a vase." Now close your eyes and envision the light of love filling your body and extending beyond your skin. Smile. Breathe the essence of the room that is being graced by the presence of the heroic goddess—you. Spiritually step into the power of your transforming shape. Breathe deeply and fully. When you open your eyes, see yourself through divine eyes.

The truth of your radiant beauty is perhaps most obvious in your partner's eyes. More likely than not, they will find your roundness sensual and erotic. Allow yourself to see through your partner's eyes and enhance your appreciation for the blossoming goddess that you are. Now is the time to stand in your sexual, creative power.

Learn to assert this power by extending your energy out to your lover and initiating lovemaking. A lot of people are reluctant to initiate sex during their partner's pregnancy because they don't want to burden you or don't want to deal with the possibility of rejection. And some people still think of obviously pregnant women as off-limits or taboo. This may sound ridiculous in the twenty-first century, but for many thousands of years, there have strict rules surrounding the physical transformation of pregnancy and childbirth. If your partner is suffering from one of the many myths regarding sex during pregnancy, be patient and have fun helping them to overcome it. In addition to being the sensual seductress that your inner goddess embodies, you can both relax and connect by creating and maintaining what we sometimes call a "love bridge."

Journeywork
The Love Bridge

For one minute each day, hold hands with your partner and silently gaze into each other's eyes. Through your silent thoughts, thank each other, say I love you, and express your love for your baby. Complete this daily practice with a heart-to-heart hug. A lot of couples enjoy doing this first thing in the morning and/or before going to sleep at night. It may feel awkward at first—you may laugh or giggle or find yourself wanting to break eye contact. Don't quit. After practicing this for a week or so, you'll forge an eye-to-eye soul connection and look forward to this special moment of silent communion with each other. Once you get past the awkward stage, don't be surprised if this moment brings tears to your eyes as your hearts open more widely to each other and the new life you're carrying.

Building and strengthening your love bridge can make a dramatic difference in your closeness and trust for each other. It is also a way to get in touch with each other's feelings and merge energy fields. Doing this will lower your stress and enhance your bond with each other because you will be regularly connecting on a deeper level. And this overwhelming love that you share not only will be felt by your baby, but it will allow you to override any sexual self-consciousness that you may be feeling.

Finding Comfortable Positions

During the first trimester, your lovemaking probably didn't change much. You could still move into all of your favorite positions with no problem. But now you'll want to make some modifications. When you're four months pregnant, you may not enjoy having sex in the missionary (man on top) position because it can be uncomfortable and in some pregnancies may not be safe. One of the best positions from this point on is on your left side with a pillow under your belly. Your aorta and vena cava are located on the right side of your body, so lying on your left side can relieve the pressure of the uterus pressing down on them. If you place your right knee on a few pillows too, your partner can more easily enter you from behind while holding you at the same time.

If you're both fans of the woman on top position, it's okay to continue using this position until the end of the fourth month. But after that, we don't recommend it. This position can put too much pressure on your hips and knees, so now's the time to try something new or revive an old favorite. You might find that being on your hands and knees, allowing your back to stretch and your belly to hang down, becomes a new favorite. This position is also renowned for stimulating the G-spot—a small, extra-sensitive area located a few inches inside your vagina on the front-facing wall.

But don't get too caught up in the technicalities. To be the best lovers you can be, make love to each other all the time, in a thousand different ways that extend into every facet of your lives together. By nurturing each other's spirits, everything else tends to fall into place.

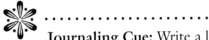

Journaling Cue: Write a love letter to your partner acknowledging them for the traits and qualities that you love and appreciate. Consider including a "love coupon" that they can redeem later.

Turning Inward

As you move through the days of your second trimester, you will likely find yourself turning inward more often. That's natural and expected because your body, mind, and spirit are in a dynamic state of flux. An important element of this honeymoon part of the journey is enjoying being alone with the baby. Enjoy that surreal floating sensation of walking on air as the baby floats inside of you. Revel in the changes you and the baby are both making, fully feeling all of the sensations and emotions that your journey brings to you. As the hero of this spiritual journey, you're the embodiment of the Goddess and are communing with the Divine within yourself and your child. There is great passion and power in this still moment at the center of the dance. Be here now.

As the weeks fly by, you and your partner will become more and more aware of the changes taking place in your body as it shifts, grows, and softens. Your sexuality also adapts to these changes—how you look, the sensations you feel within and without. Be consciously aware of them and rejoice in them! The life inside you invites your continuing amazement and curiosity, as each day—each week—brings something new.

As you practice communing with the baby and centering yourself, you will continue to grow in your connection with one another. That said, there will be times when you just aren't up for connecting with anyone, including the one inside of you. That's okay. It's perfectly normal to want some "me" time, and we encourage you to give yourself a break and be gentle with yourself. Go to that still center and ask your soul what you need to be replenished, calmed, soothed, and refreshed. These little hiatuses can be beneficial for you, your baby, and for your partner. Everyone can use a little alone time.

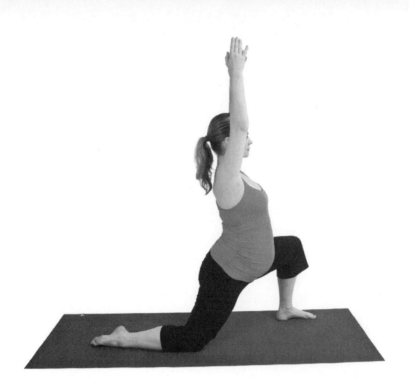

Yoga Pose
Crescent Lunge
Strengthening

This pose will help to keep your internal flame bright and your circulation strong. Lunges help open your heart and hips. They create more space for breathing and can decrease the pain of sciatica. Lunges also build strength in your core and your thighs, which will be important throughout your pregnancy and for pushing when you're giving birth. Lunging with your arms outstretched also builds strength in your arms and shoulders, preparing you to carry your bundle of joy after they are born.

To move into the lunge, begin on your hands and knees.

Bring your thumbs together.

Step your left foot to the outside of your left hand.

Bring your hands, one at a time, to your left thigh.

Make sure your knee stays directly over the ankle and the top of the right foot stays down on the ground.

Either stay here lunging forward or curl your right toes under and lift your right knee off of the ground. As you inhale, lengthen your upper torso by gently lifting your rib cage. As you exhale, slowly press your stomach muscles inward toward your spine.

After you have completed the crescent lunge on your left leg, switch legs and do it with your right leg.

Optional: Lift your arms and lengthen your upper body as if an invisible string is attached to the top of your head, pulling up your body.

Note: Take care not to lunge too deeply and over-stretch your hips.

If you feel comfortable, hold this pose for a few full breaths or a little longer.

Repeat with the opposite leg.

Benefits

- Strengthens and tones legs.

- Increases balance.

- Side lunge can help turn an occiput posterior baby, alleviating back pain, or can help an asynclitic baby to turn and descend by opening up one side of the pelvis at a time.

Precautions

- The main concern with lunges is overstretching and creating instability or pain in the hip or lower abdomen, where the ligaments attach to the uterus.

- The other caution is that as the baby grows and gets heavier, the weight on the knees needs to be monitored. Especially in the third trimester, if the back knee is off the ground, as in a crescent lunge, it is best to keep one or both hands on the front thigh and lift one at a time slowly to make sure the knee can take the weight easily and without pain.

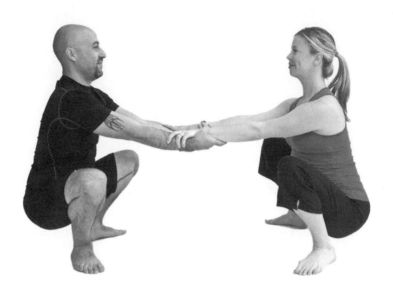

Yoga Pose
Squatting
Strengthening

To practice the squatting pose, stand facing your partner with your feet a little wider than hip-width apart. Angle your feet so that your toes are slightly turned out.

Hold hands with your partner and, while keeping your feet flat on the floor, slowly bend your knees, moving into a squat position. Make sure your legs are spread wide enough to provide space for your belly.

While holding this position, practice strengthening your pelvic floor muscles by engaging and releasing them. This Kegel exercise is very important for women who have had babies prior to the present pregnancy because the muscles that support your bladder and other internal organs in the pelvic region can become weak.

Practice and get comfortable with the squatting pose, particularly if you plan to use this pose during labor and delivery.

Benefits

Practicing this pose will strengthen your legs, back, and core muscles and stretch the muscles and tendons around your hips. Practiced several times a week, this pose will prepare you to deliver while squatting.

Squatting is one of the best positions for labor and childbirth because it can:

- speed the progress of labor

- relieve back pain

- help the pelvic opening to increase by up to 30 percent versus lying on your back

- reduce pushing time

Precautions

- This pose is not recommended if you are in danger of or have been experiencing preterm labor.

- This pose is not advised if you are in labor and the baby is high in the pelvis. If the baby is low enough, this position helps the baby move down the birth canal because of the pressure the legs put on the belly.

- This pose can be quite intense if done during a contraction before the pushing phase. It is best to do it between contractions or during pushing.

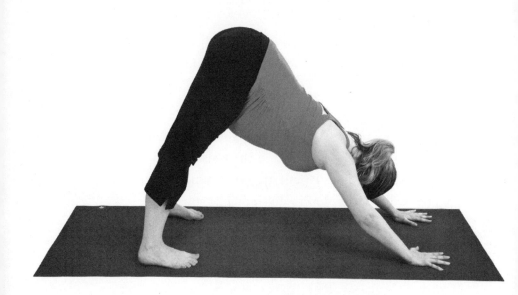

Yoga Pose
Downward-Facing Dog
Energy and Clarity

To move into downward-facing dog, start on your hands and knees. Curl your toes under and lift your knees off the ground, straightening your legs.

Bring your chest toward your thighs and make an upside-down V with your body. Your feet should be hip-width apart or wider as your belly gets bigger.

Stay here for one to three breaths.

Benefits
- Great for fatigue.

- Helps relieve leg and back pain.

- Stretches shoulders and shoulder blades, arms, hamstrings, lower back, and calves.

- Relaxes the lower uterine area to make it more symmetrical.

Precautions
- Some days it may not feel good, so skip it on those days.

- If your hamstrings and lower back are tight, you may not be able to flatten your feet on the ground. Tiptoes are fine, and bending your knees is also acceptable.

- Contraindicated if you are experiencing heartburn or in third trimester and have a large amount of amniotic fluid.

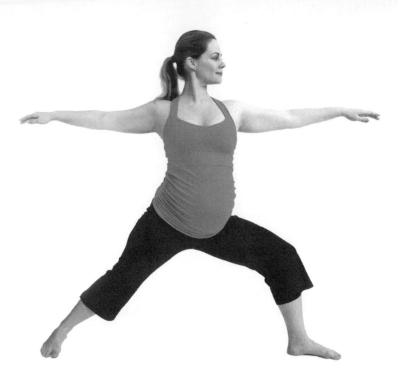

Yoga Pose
Warrior II
Powerful Opening

Beginning in Warrior I (see page 65), open the arms out to the side, lengthening them in opposite directions. You will be pulled in many directions as a new mom, and this pose is a metaphor for how flexible you can become and also how open your heart will be to this new baby.

Turn the back foot so that it's perpendicular to your front foot.

Keep your front knee bent. Notice how it feels to be grounded in this posture and the power it evokes. This pose calls to mind the softness and power of pregnancy and motherhood, and it teaches you to simultaneously experience this power and openness.

Benefits
- Increases your stability and grounds you to Mother Earth.
- Enhances your awareness of the softness and power of pregnancy and motherhood.

Precautions
- As your baby grows, your own center of gravity will change. Be sure you are feeling balanced when you practice this pose.
- Hold this position only for as long as it feels steady and comfortable.

As you complete your second trimester, you also complete the initiation stage of your epic journey. You have passed the tests and weathered the difficulties of pregnancy for six months now, and you continue to prevail. You've undergone a significant emotional, physical, and spiritual transformation, and you've no doubt had a few heart-to-heart talks with yourself about how you want this pregnancy to proceed and what sort of mother you want to be. You're probably used to the healthy changes that you've made and are even embracing them now. Everything is proceeding right on schedule, and you are ready and prepared for the next stage of your journey.

Part 3
Third Trimester

Approaching the Inmost Cave

On your hero's journey, the inmost cave represents the space where the treasure is hidden. The more precious the treasure, the more challenges the hero encounters in the quest to retrieve it. During this time of physical and spiritual expansion, you will feel your strength and your will being tested. Physically, your baby is growing and pushing on your internal organs, causing shortness of breath, varicose veins, sleeplessness, and restless leg syndrome. Hormonal fluctuations and other changes, along with the baby's added weight, are moving you beyond the daydreaming phase of having a child into the real deal: the place where your challenges actually change you—and you experience an expansion into someone greater than you were before, a mother capable of creating, birthing, and nurturing new life.

As you venture deeper into the cave, you enter a metaphysical space that shamans and religious philosophers call a liminal state of being; that is, an in-between place that is neither in this world nor in the spirit world but is standing on the threshold. The word *liminal* comes from the Latin word that means "a threshold." This middle space is the matrix of creation; it's where the powers of spirit intermingle with the hopes and intentions of this world to produce miracles. In this case, the miracle is the tiny being growing inside you, and by attuning yourself to its existence, you touch the veil that is said to separate spirit from human form. This journey is now bringing you closer to what lies beyond the veil.

Third Trimester:
What's Happening?

Month Seven
Physically

- The baby's eyelids open, and they can now see and respond to light outside the womb.

- The baby can also respond to touch and sound.

- The baby's arms and legs are gaining length and strength, making punches and kicks more vigorous.

- The cells lining the air sacs in the baby's lungs begin secreting a substance that keeps them inflated. This is an important development that prepares the baby for breathing outside of your womb.

- The baby gains at least 1 pound, and you gain 3 to 5 pounds.

Spiritually

As the baby's ability to respond to touch, light, and sound increases, you can increase your communication and begin to learn more about each other. As your communication becomes more physical, be sure to continue to develop the spirit-to-spirit connection that you've formed with your baby through your silent thoughts and emotions. Many women say they feel particularly dreamy during this month and find great pleasure in silently communing with the spirit of their baby simply by feeling the love they already share with one another.

Month Eight

Physically

- The baby can blink their eyes in reaction to outside light.

- The baby's fat doubles, smoothing out some of the wrinkles and creating a softer appearance. This rounding out helps the baby's body to regulate temperature after birth.

- Hiccups are common for the baby during this month. They may feel like sudden jerks to you, but they are normal and don't hurt the baby or you.

- As the baby's brain rapidly grows, they will start to dream. During this month and from this point forward, the baby will have REM (rapid eye movement/dream-stage sleep) and non-REM sleep stages.

- Baby may turn to a head-down position around the thirty-fourth week of your pregnancy.

- By the end of this month, baby is 16 to 18 inches long and weighs 3 to 4 pounds.

Spiritually

During this month, women often report having vivid dreams about their babies. We don't think it's a coincidence that this is also the month when the baby begins to dream. There are many stories of babies communicating important messages to their mothers through dreams. Now is the time to sink into your intuitive mind and gut instincts. Many women enjoy keeping a dream journal during this time. You can also experiment by writing down questions that you want to ask while you're dreaming and by giving yourself the command to remember your dreams.

Month Nine

Physically

- The baby is piling on fat during this final month in preparation for his or her entry into the world.

- The baby is breathing, sucking a thumb, turning the head, and practicing motor skills like opening and closing hands, reaching, pulling, pushing, and sometimes punching.

- As the baby runs out of room in your uterus, they will spend most of the time curled up like a little ball, but you will still be able to feel movement.

- At the time of delivery, the baby will likely weigh between 6 and 8 pounds and be 19 to 21 inches tall.

Spiritually

As the baby physically curls up inside your womb, you may find yourself curling up emotionally and becoming more quiet and introspective. Now is the time to give your inner voice center stage. Consciously dismiss the mind chatter of the inner critic, the worrier, or any other voices that compete for your attention. Some women say that they lapse into long, silent dialogs with their babies. These quiet moments help to weave the spiritual bond that is eternal between mother and child.

Chapter 5

The Path of Expansion

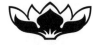

Once your baby arrives, the world
is no more the same than you are.
Because from our very bodies we add
to the collective human destiny.

Claire Fontaine,
Have Mother, Will Travel

Your body and your baby are expanding, and you're enduring the challenges of this expansion. At the start of the third trimester, your baby is about an inch long and weighs up to three pounds. The thin coat of fine hair covering the baby is shedding. The baby is also practicing breathing, sometimes perceptibly. Your baby's hearing is fully developed, and they can respond to the soothing sound of your voice as you talk, hum, or sing directly to them.

By now, you'll be looking more and more like those pregnant, glowing celebrities on the covers of magazines. Surges of hormones will make your skin and hair gleam. Many women find their hair and nails grow longer and stronger than ever before. You'll also begin to take on the womanly contours of those ancient fertility figures—larger breasts, belly heavy with child. You may now have an additional two pounds of breast tissue, and as birth gets closer you may see that your nipples are leaking colostrum, the fluid that feeds baby in the first weeks of life. You're also putting on weight; some of it is the baby's and some yours (don't worry about this, but stay on the nutrition and exercise program your medical team have advised).

Other new sensations throughout the third trimester include the famous Braxton Hicks contractions, the false labor or practice cramping named after John Braxton Hicks, an English physician, who identified them in the 1870s. These contractions, which can be brought on by dehydration or a full bladder, can be relieved by emptying your bladder, movement, lying down on your left side, or by rhythmic breathing. They're nature's way of giving you a practice run for the real thing.

As the third trimester goes on, the baby gains weight, changes position, and tends to move into a head-down position to begin the process of birth. By the last month of the third trimester, baby will be almost twenty inches long and nearly seven pounds. Their eyes will be able to open and close and see light through your belly. Not only that, the little hands and feet that you saw on your ultrasound are moving. Hands can grasp and feet (as you'll know) are kicking often.

Meanwhile, even as your baby is growing in ways that make them more physically independent from you, your bond—emotionally, spiritually, and psychologically—is deepening. Metaphorically, as you move toward the inmost cave during the third trimester, you're consciously choosing to face and conquer your fears, letting your old sense of self fall away and expanding beyond the boundaries of who you formerly were. No longer is your identity solely about you; your baby is now becoming a part of who you are—a separate person who is nevertheless eternally connected through the sacred bond of mother and child. Your inner sense of divinity will grow to help you meet the challenge of reimagining yourself. While your body shifts and changes in ways that are sometimes uncomfortable, you will become more and more aware of your co-creative role, working in tandem with your higher power to bring forth new life.

 . . . .

Journaling Cue: Take a few minutes to reflect on the previous paragraph. Then write a letter to your inner sense of divinity, sharing your thoughts, posing questions, or simply saying thank you.

Body and Spirit at the Threshold

As you approach the inmost cave, your sense of identity may feel as though it's beginning to dissolve. The fear of losing who you are can bring about disorientation. You have begun a period of transition where normal limits of self-understanding are relaxed. Although the challenges on this path can be difficult, the changes can lead to what poet William Blake called "a higher innocence," by which he meant a transformational state of enlightenment. As your body and your identity are challenged, you discover the possibilities of expanding your limits: physical, psychological, and spiritual.

As you stand on the threshold of motherhood, you are standing as three women: yourself before pregnancy, the dual self you are now (with two beings sharing one body), and your newly reborn self as the giver of life to a newborn baby. This threshold allows you the opportunity to tap into divine energy. By opening your heart to the loving light of the spirit realm, you grow stronger, wiser, and more centered, literally becoming an en*light*-ened mother.

When the expectant mother moves into the third trimester, many world cultures view this as a magical state of being. In numerous ancient legends, pregnant woman are considered more powerful than even the best medicine man or shaman. This is, in part, because the mother-to-be becomes a person who is between heaven and earth, and consequently has the power of both. In Celtic myth, people in this state have the ability to see fairies and other powerful spirits. Poets are considered "spirit walkers" in Celtic lore because they have the godlike power of the word yet are not gods. These abilities are essential for the hero as she walks toward the inmost cave. Your mother's intuition is developing. Insight and the ability to tap into guidance from your higher self will help you overcome the challenges of this stage. When you finish on this path, not only will you be stronger, you will retain the essence of these abilities to guide you on through motherhood.

Your inner changes are mirrored by outer changes in your body, and you may begin to feel like the ugly duckling or the princess who must kiss the frog before she can live happily ever after. Swans and frogs are considered powerful beings in European folklore because they transform and live in an in-between state. Ugly ducklings mature into swans; frogs traverse the worlds of water and land, bringing wisdom from the other side. Perhaps this is why both frogs and swans have been considered totem animals for fertility, love, and childbearing in many world cultures, including the Celtic and ancient Egyptian cultures. Totem animals are special beings that connect us to the wisdom of both nature and the spirit world.

Meditating on these totem animals, the swan and the frog, will help you to accept that physically you are no longer the person you were before you conceived. You can't do some of the things you used to do. You may have started eating differently, foregoing that glass of wine at dinner, and taking special care of your body with vitamins and exercise. Your old clothes don't fit. You can't play some of your favorite sports and may not even fit comfortably behind the wheel of your car! You might have trouble sleeping and have to make frequent trips to the bathroom. Your body is transforming, and although you may be having fears that things will never be the same, the swan teaches you to stay focused on the beautiful being that you are becoming.

The frog can also be your guide as the challenges of the third trimester unfold. It embodies the fluid, transitional nature of water, which represents spirit, reminding you to let a higher power move you. The frog also lives on land, showing the importance of staying grounded and connected to the earth. This duality of water/spirit and land/earth is a mirror to your experience. Here on your journey, you are bringing spirit through your body, where the very elements of the earth come together in your womb to create new life. The myth of the frog prince teaches that embracing the liminal state by kissing the frog will transform it into your prince—your prize gift of a new baby. You might consider wearing a swan and/or frog totem as jewelry or creating a small shrine to your "becoming" self with images of these animals as a way to internalize the changes taking place in you and to honor your own transformation.

Transforming Challenge into Change

The transitional state presents an opportunity for great transformation, but the price is fully letting go of your former self. In the myths of most world cultures, the abandonment of one's old ego is portrayed as the hero's descent into a dark place often described as the underworld, a wilderness, a desert, or a wide expanse of sea. These settings are always filled with monsters and demons, which represent the struggle to change and the parts of yourself that may be afraid or resistant to letting go of who you used to be.

In Buddhism, Prince Siddhartha came to this place at the point in his journey when he was closest to enlightenment. Siddhartha was meditating under a tree when the demon Mara (a word that literally means death) came and challenged him. Mara sent monsters, fire, storms, and winds to move Siddhartha from his task of finding enlightenment, but Siddhartha sat still through all of it. Mara claimed that the seat of enlightenment belonged to him, and his monster army cried out their assent as witnesses. Siddhartha quietly touched the earth, which responded that he was the rightful owner of the place of peace and understanding. Mara then vanished, and Siddhartha became the Buddha—the enlightened one. In this story Mara stands for the ego, which must pass away in favor of the light of a new self-understanding. Although the circumstances are fearful and menacing, Siddhartha knows that his ego must disappear before he can attain enlightenment. By touching the ground, he roots himself to the earth, which sends him life-giving energy to sustain this challenge.

It is important to stay grounded during this transitional time. Descending into the dark reaches of oneself and forging a new identity are great challenges. The story of the Buddha's enlightenment teaches the hero to find a calm spiritual center that will give you strength on the path of challenge and expansion. Yoga is one way to do this. Even the Buddha studied yoga as part of his meditation practice. Spending some time each day doing the yoga poses in this book can be a great support to you now, helping to clear your mind, ease your body, and bring you into a centered state. Let the Buddha inspire you to touch the earth by meditating on the Earth Mother inside of you and letting her arise within your spirit to create a higher version of yourself—a stronger person who is able to cross this threshold. This is important for you now and may play a role in your future too. Research indicates that a mother's distress and depression can affect the sleeping patterns of her baby *after* they are born.

Affecting Baby's Sleep Patterns

A 1998 study by Armstrong and colleagues set out to see if maternal distress and depression could change or affect childhood sleep problems after the baby was born. This study discovered something groundbreaking: childhood sleep problems may have their beginnings in the prenatal period, or in the womb. From this work they decided that mothers at risk for excessive anxiety or depression during pregnancy should have an extensive workup and possible therapy because of the potential this process could have on the fetus. Cindy-Lee Dennis (associate professor at the Lawrence S. Bloomberg Faculty of Nursing, University of Toronto) and Lori Ross (Centre for Addiction and Mental Health, Toronto, ON) replicated these findings in 2005, when they discovered mothers who exhibited depression between weeks four and eight of their pregnancy had babies that woke more between 10 PM and 6 AM. These studies are meant not to scare you but to illustrate how your behavior can change the climate of your baby's internal world in the uterus.

For example, baby may be patterning his wake and sleep times with yours. There is more research needed in this area, but many of our patients who are early risers have babies who are early risers, and many of the mothers who stayed up late had babies who wanted to stay up late. This might make a case for pregnant women to improve sleep hygiene by going to bed at a reasonable hour and getting eight or more hours of quality sleep. We know this is easier said than done, but we believe it's one of the most important things that you can do for you and the baby.

The Near-Life Experience

At this point, you are probably beginning to see that pregnancy, with its ever-changing presence, gives you tremendous power. As you grow closer to the time of birth, we want to bring up a concept that we believe has great significance for the hero's path of challenge and expansion: the near-*life* experience.

You are probably familiar with the idea of the near-death experience, where people come close to dying and then see a white light, a tunnel, and their deceased relatives. The loved ones (or angels) tell them to go back to earth, and they return to their bodies completely transformed by the experience. These people often relate a new sense of their mission in life and of living with new conviction and strength.

We believe that the pregnant woman goes through a similar experience when she is in labor. It begins during the trimesters leading up to birth, when she is connecting with the world of the unborn through meditation, fetal heart connection, and other methods we've already discussed. As obstetricians, we have personally witnessed the ecstasy—the "high," if you will—of a new mother giving birth. Part of this is the mixture of chemicals the body produces during labor, but there is also something more sublime. In the altered state of consciousness that takes place while delivering the baby, the mother comes into direct contact with the miracle of life, not only as a witness but as an active participant. The fact that your body, mind, and spirit are hosting a new life brings you closer to merging with the Divine. Just as the near-death experience brings a renewed feeling of connectedness, the near-life experience does the same. When you reach this point in your journey, you can look back on everything you experienced while walking the path of challenge and expansion and know that you've received blessed gifts: not only your child but also the new strength, conviction, and confidence in your ability to be a mother.

 . . . .

Journaling Cue: Reflect on your journey up to this point. What were the highlights? What has surprised you? What were the pains? How have these experiences served you as the hero of this journey? What have you learned?

Communicating with Your Baby Using Light

By month seven, the baby can detect light and darkness and possibly see silhouettes outside the womb. When our friend Sylvia brought her baby home, her Siamese cat, Sheba, jumped up on the bed to check out Ben out. Sylvia thought Ben would be startled, but instead he started to happily squirm and smile. It's possible that Ben recognized Sheba's shape as familiar. Sylvia told us that when she was pregnant, Sheba would often parade back and forth on the windowsill while she was meditating or would curl up on her belly. Of course, there's no way to know if that's why Ben had an immediately positive response to Sheba, but we're inclined to believe the familiar silhouette theory.

Connecting Deeper
Through the Elements

The journeywork in this book and the spiritual amplification you'll feel while doing our yoga exercises are tools to develop your spiritual muscles. These spiritual muscles will help you to forge a deeper near-birth bonding with your baby. In the following physical and psychological exercises for your "near-life" third trimester, we have chosen the elements—earth, air, fire, and water—as the basis of your journeywork. Divided into four sections, there are exercises for each element, collectively the basis of all life on earth.

Journeywork
Earth

The ground is your source at a very elemental level, and you are rooted to it for sustenance and support. The body is carbon based and the earth is carbon based. We start from the earth and return to the earth. Here we present an earth meditation where you simply lie upon the ground and allow your skin to touch the earth as you sense its natural rhythmic pulsations.

Connect with the earth underneath you. Go to a safe place in nature and lie on your left side, allowing your bare pregnant belly to touch the ground. Allow you and the baby to be supported by the earth. If the baby is moving, envision their little feet pushing against the earth through your belly.

Another option is walking a labyrinth or engaging in a walking meditation where with every footstep you repeat the name of your unborn baby; if there is no name yet, then choose another mantra that fits. Also look at your connection with the earth via the foods that you eat. You receive vital elements like magnesium, calcium, and iron from the food you consume; this food is provided to you by the sun, water, and by the earth itself.

Journeywork
Air

Breath is essential for life. In the same way that oxygen is formed from two molecules (as in O_2), the mother and baby are two separate cosmic molecules functioning as one. In Sanskrit, *prana* means vital life, or breath; in Ayurveda, the traditional medicine of India, prana enters the body through your breath and goes to every cell in your body.

This exercise will harmonize you and your baby through the breath of life. You will be guiding your breath through your lungs and circulatory system and into your baby, and then the baby will give you its waste and carbon dioxide to exhale. Remember, you are currently one unit functioning as two beings.

Bring yourself either into a sitting position or lie on your left side with a pillow placed between your knees. The goal here is to be as comfortable and weightless as possible.

Focus on your breath. This very breath, right now, will soon be the oxygen that feeds your baby.

Relax your belly and take in a deep breath.

With the next breath, imagine this oxygen filling your lungs and entering your heart.

With the next breath, imagine this oxygen traveling into your bloodstream and heading downward, toward your belly. Once in the aorta, the blood will pump toward your uterine arteries and begin filling the uterus with this oxygen-rich connection.

Imagine the uterus as light and energy, warm and pulsating. The pulsations are coming from you, and they are surrounding your baby with the sound of your heart and the sense of your love.

With the next breath, allow the oxygen to pulsate into the placenta, filling it with the same love and warmth. Imagine the placenta filling with each individual breath.

When the placenta is full of love, energy, and oxygen, allow it to pass into the umbilical vein coursing toward the baby.

As the umbilical vein fills with oxygen-rich blood, notice how it bypasses the baby's lungs (as this breath comes from you) and proceeds to your baby's heart—the heart that you created. This little heart is able to receive your oxygen-rich gift and send it throughout the baby's body.

As the baby's body uses the oxygen and love you have sent, allow the baby to let go of carbon dioxide and other wastes and give them to you. Let your baby know you want this, and surround it with the acceptance that you are taking care of everything as only a mother can do.

This blood now courses into the umbilical arteries by the pumping of the baby's heart in cadence with yours as it enters the placenta. With your next exhalation, imagine that blood crossing the placenta and entering your vena cava (the largest vein in the body, bringing blood to and from the heart to be oxygenated and then circulated) on its way back to your heart. This blood carries the elements and traces of your baby; this blood has touched every one of your baby's cells.

Once in the heart, this blood now pumps into the lungs, and on the very next exhale feel the breath that has been inside your baby. Notice how every breath has the scent of your child and the connection between the two of you. Allow yourself to stay in this place until you're done, and then slowly open your eyes and realize you are always in contact with your little one.

Journeywork
Fire

Its flames are synonymous with the heat and pulsation of the blood. Fire is a cleansing element that is also associated with the raw, unpredictable power that can be translated to labor. Fire is unpredictable, like the hormones that are powerful messengers flowing through your blood. The blood itself being red and rich with oxygen carries vital power to the baby through the placenta and umbilical cord.

A special ceremony involving the unpredictability of fire is allowing the flames to consume your fears. There is unpredictability to becoming a mother, whether for the first or the fourth time. Take time to write those fears on separate pieces of paper; after writing them down, place them in a paper bag and close them up, sealing them away from you forever. If you have a fireplace or an outdoor grill, use this to safely burn this bag of fears, watching its smoke rise into the atmosphere. Envision those fears dissipating.

Journeywork
Water

Water, considered to be the element of the mother of us all by many African religions, is a wonderful support for the mother during her spiritual pregnancy. As a species we are born from water, and when we are pre-fetuses, we even look something like little tadpoles. In fact, according to African-American folklore, when a woman dreams of fish, it means she or someone she knows is pregnant. The remnants of these ancient beliefs remind us of the significance of water as the life-giving origin of our species.

The water of the womb is amniotic fluid. Your baby is supported in a weightless, waterlike environment, and the fluid is just as essential as the oxygen for development. Plasma makes up the matrix for the red and white blood cells, and we all need water to survive. Your baby is a little reverse scuba diver, breathing amniotic fluid late in the second trimester when he or she expands that little set of new lungs. By staying well hydrated during your pregnancy, you can increase amniotic fluid since what you drink will go through to your baby. If you increase your fluid volume, your baby will urinate more and add to its own amniotic fluid.

If you have the benefit of a heated pool or a hot tub, you can warm the water to 99 degrees and submerge yourself in the warmth of the weightless water. Feel what your baby feels in this warm environment provided by your warmth and love. You might like to work with the imagery of the Yoruba mother goddess Yemaya, who watches over pregnant women and helps the embryo develop into a healthy baby. You can surround yourself with her favorite colors of white and blue and bring ocean shells and blue glass to the edges of your tub. Envision that universal cycle of motherhood enveloping your baby as it once surrounded you. Know that you are connected across the sacred waters to the eons of mothers who have come before you.

You are walking the same sacred path as your ancestors—the same path that your children will walk someday. This part of your journey calls to mind classic scenes from sacred pilgrimages. Have you ever seen images of pilgrims on the path to a sacred place walking on their knees or barefoot? And yet, if you talk to these pilgrims at this point in their pilgrimage—just before they reach their sacred goal—they are usually ecstatic. An inner joy takes over them (what runners sometimes call their "second wind"), and that spiritual expansion moves them toward their finish line.

As your body and the body of the child within you evolve in dynamic co-creation, your awareness changes, expands, and begins to awaken to a new self—your new identity as a mother. You are now getting pretty good at transforming challenge into change, including altering your sleep cycle to help condition your baby for life after birth. You have a new appreciation for the near- life experience and are becoming more grounded in your role of mother. By continuing to connect with the baby and Spirit through the elements, you can maintain your sense of inner and outer balance. This is essential because your body is concentrating its energy, focus, blood, and tissue to build the most transcendental thing in the world—a new life.

Chapter 6

The Journey's Crowning

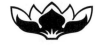

Toward the end of your third trimester, you will have spent about half a year becoming a mother-to-be, a journey with many miracle mileposts and intimations of the miracle about to be born. The last trimester, while challenging, is also a time of joy. Your baby's birth is crowning the horizon, signaling the culmination of your spiritual pregnancy journey. Light is coming into the picture quite literally. Your baby opens their eyes in the third trimester and begins to see shapes, outlines, and light.

We talked about the unpleasant effects that your growing baby has on your energy, but midwives also call the end of the third trimester the "lightening" because the movement of the baby downward relieves pressure on your breathing. You'll feel the baby moving, stretching, and expanding every day. By the time you're ready to give birth, you can expect your weight to increase by up to thirty-five pounds. Some of this is due to the baby's weight and some is placenta, amniotic fluid, increased blood and fluids, and extra fat stores.

Preparing for Physical Separation

As the hero, soon you will reach into the spiritual infinite and bring your own Holy Grail into the world. So it's no surprise that the third trimester is sometimes wrought with emotional ups and downs. And just as you start to get really excited about the special day approaching, you may also start to feel sad. As the child within you prepares to live in the outside world, there's a natural feeling of melancholy, which can deepen after pregnancy. This is commonly referred to as the baby blues, while more serious conditions are called post-partum depression. Much has been written about this, but from the spiritual perspective, when you create a new life within your body, you touch a divine realm. Now, as the channel between you and the infinite begins to close and you return to a more regular existence, it makes sense that this separation may be accompanied by a feeling of loss.

If you can begin to understand the dynamic of separation and the process of coming back to the real world before the actual birth occurs, you can prepare yourself for a smoother transition from pregnancy to motherhood. The first step is to meditate on your baby becoming their own person even while they are connected to you in the womb. Your baby spends a lot of time sucking their thumb now, practicing for nursing. Fingers and toes are all differentiated, and their eyes are open much of the time. Your baby is beginning to turn their attention from the light of the spirit realm to the light of the physical realm.

This time of growing differentiation of baby from mother is a perfect time to explore the spiritual concept of light. The first movements of creation in the Judeo-Christian Bible are heralded by the phrase "let there be light." As explained so memorably in the film *Under the Tuscan Sun,* the Italian translation of "to give birth" is *dare alla luce,* or "to give to the light." When you give birth, you give light to light. Exercises such as the following one, together with a deepened spiritual awareness of this process, should help ease any anxieties as your miraculous creation begins to individuate from you and prepares to bring his or her own distinctive light into the world.

Journeywork
Lighting Up the Womb

One way to process the emotional understanding of your baby's separateness is by meditating and working with the baby's perception of light. Beginning at about week twenty-eight, your baby's eyesight is developing, and they can blink. Baby can perceive a flashlight moved across your belly as a red or orange light. When you play with light over your belly, you'll most likely feel the baby move to avoid the light since it is a foreign and unfamiliar sensation. Practice showing your baby the movement of light accompanied by soothing sounds of encouragement to see if that changes the pattern of movement. As you do this, you can be assured that your baby's eyes are beginning to strengthen and follow the light.

Our patient Marci turned the light on and off several times in a row to see if her baby would respond. At eight months, he responded by kicking her. From that point on, it became a game that they played. When Kim was born and Marci projected the flashing light on the inside of her crib, Kim would kick as he had in the womb.

Many birthing procedures are now using darkened rooms so that babies do not have to go from the soft shadow world of the womb into the blinding light of an operating room beacon. As you play with light and your baby shifts within you, imagine the light gradually increasing until it envelops them in a warm (but not blinding) luminosity. Imagine that light surrounding both of you as the baby moves to separate from you and take their place in that light.

Spiritual Cleansing and the Nesting Instinct

As your journey takes you closer to your day of birthing, your instinct to prepare the nest will lead you to complete your decorating or preparations in the nursery and elsewhere in the house. Nature's instincts are there for a reason. New mothers of all species experience a phenomenon called "the nesting instinct."

Most commonly, this happens in the last part of third trimester as the new mother begins to feel that the pregnancy is moving toward completion. In the first two trimesters, much of your journey was about going inward. Now you turn outward, back into the real world, to prepare for baby's arrival. Your home becomes a nest, and you may find yourself spending a lot of time feathering that nest: making sure it's clean, bright, and nurturing. Follow your instincts and intuition, and make the act of creating the nest a sacred process.

Ancient traditions teach that consecrating one's space is essential when bringing new life into one's home. Renewed vitality is recognized as a daily gift to be welcomed and celebrated in rituals that follow the cycle of the sun from morning to night. These practices continue across the globe, and you can embrace them as a guide for your nesting instincts. For instance, in Bali, where space clearing is a deeply spiritual practice, every morning, all over cities and mountain villages, people come out in front of their houses and whisk the ground clean with stiff, hand-held brooms. The whisking not only drives away bad spirits and dirt, it also refreshes the energy of the home. In your case it can symbolically create a fertile ground for a new seed to take root within your family.

Journeywork
Sacred Cleansing

You can incorporate the Balinese practice into your sacred cleansing process by searching craft markets for a whisk broom made of natural fibers. Adorn your whisk with ribbons and items that represent the beginning of a new life in your home. You might choose to attach a treasured piece of jewelry from a beloved ancestor whom you invite to watch over your infant. Or you might add colorful trinkets that represent newborn babies: booties, a baby locket, even a baby charm bracelet. What's most important is that your broom reflects your feelings of love for your baby. As you furnish your baby's room, find a special place to rest your broom as a symbol that this space will remain cleansed and ready to receive fresh energy. Set an intention for the room and the entire house to become a safe, welcoming environment for your little one.

Consider drawing upon the traditional Chinese practice of feng shui, which embraces space clearing as part of creating harmonious vibrations for luck, love, health and safety. In feng shui, clutter and disorder invite bad or negative chi, or energy flow. Now is the time to give away or discard anything that isn't useful, beautiful, or positive in some way. Let your nesting instinct guide you through your home and notice belongings that energize you versus those items that seem stuck in the past. Perhaps there are things that represent old chapters in your life, and you are ready to part with them. If possible, empty the closet in your baby's room of everything except new gifts for them. If the baby will share your room, make a symbolic space for their belongings, whether that's a new dresser or trunk. And be sure to clear your bed of clutter, both underneath and around it. You might even hire a professional organizer or feng shui expert.

Feng shui not only offers important insights into clearing space for your baby, it also suggests activities that can help you as you crown your pregnancy journey. Facing the head of your bed in the north or east direction is said to help improve the quality of sleep—a challenge often faced by women in the third trimester. Surround yourself with colors that add vitality and health to your home: pink, green, indigo, and red. Paint is a wonderful way to introduce these colors to you and your baby's space, but remember to choose nontoxic, low-VOC paints. An alternative is to drape soft, colorful fabrics from the walls, ceilings, or windows, or incorporate color through your home accessories. It is said that red can help increase appetite, so use it judiciously in the kitchen and dining room to improve appetites diminished by morning sickness and fatigue. Try ringing bells (Balinese bells or singing bowls are known for their space-cleansing properties) or playing peaceful music to introduce positive vibrations and chase out stagnant energy. These sounds will also have a calming effect on you.

Doing a formal spiritual cleansing ceremony (called space clearing) is another way to ready your nest that offers many benefits. In her book *Creating Sacred Space with Feng Shui*, Karen Kingston, one of the best-known Western practitioners of this Balinese tradition, describes a twenty-one-step space-clearing ceremony that includes creating flower offerings, setting up an altar, and clapping out stagnant energy.[31] She believes that while giving your home a spiritual cleansing is a healthy and positive way to nest before the baby comes, the energies released during the ceremony can be too strong for the baby, so it's important that pregnant or nursing mothers are not present during a formal ceremony. A professional can be retained for this process, or friends and relatives can learn to do the ceremony on your behalf. It's a perfect opportunity to take a "me day" to relax outside of the home: get a manicure, take a walk in the sun, and think positive thoughts while loved ones cleanse your home.

 . . . .

Journaling Cue: While you are on your "me day," give some thought to your behaviors and habits. Write down one or two behaviors or habits that you know you would be better off without but can't seem to give up. Write down ten ways that giving up each of these behaviors can benefit you and your baby.

As your hero's journey moves toward completion, the idea of homecoming becomes imminent. Whether you're birthing at home or will be returning home after birthing, it will be a newly transformed place—a nest infused with spiritual blessings and ready to cradle a new life. Some women like to have a spiritual teacher or religious advisor come to the house to bless it before their baby comes home for the first time.

Many religions have home-blessing traditions. In Hindu culture, to invite the gods and their positive attributes, offerings are made, candles are lit, and prayers are said. Shinto rituals in Japan entail hand clapping to let the gods know you have arrived. Your religious or spiritual tradition will also have its own rituals of home blessing, which can be a rich experience for you during this stage. Becoming mindful of the divine presence in your home will ease your transition from hosting a new spirit in your body to birthing it into the world. As you complete this trimester, revel in the knowledge that you're surrounded and embraced by an ever-present loving energy. The home blessing is a wonderful way to reaffirm this truth.

The Name Game

Whether you know if your baby is a girl or a boy or not, by now you've probably compiled a list of potential names. As your sense of your baby's personhood grows stronger, some of the names may no longer seem to fit, while others may rise to the top of the list. As you move steadily toward being baby and you, instead of baby *in* you, the ritual of naming is on the horizon. When you name your child, you also gain a new name for yourself, much as the spiritual warriors in global folklore took on a new name after their journeys. Your new name is Mom, Mummy, Mama, or any of the variations on that magical name of Mother. Your offspring must also be gifted with a name that embodies their essence and identifies a place in this world.

World cultures have elaborate ceremonies and customs around the naming of a child. These traditions acknowledge the transitional nature of a baby's passage from the womb, with its doorway to the infinite behind the child and its doorway to the physical realm ahead. The selection of a name marks the significance of this individuated little person as he or she steps through the doorway ahead and into the light of physical being. Beliefs from around the globe may inspire you with rituals for honoring your baby with a name.

In Christian cultures, baptism was usually the naming ceremony where parents introduced their child to the world at large and gave them their names along with their godparents. Orthodox Christians in the Eastern tradition had a special naming ceremony eight days after the child's birth. An ancient practice called "churching" was also practiced, which meant that the new mother needed to cleanse herself and come to church afterwards with her baby for prayer. Today, these ancient practices continue along with secular naming ceremonies that have arisen amongst those who aren't religious but understand the sacred significance of granting a child their name.

In the Jewish tradition, a child's Jewish name connects them to the Jewish nation as a whole. Baby boys are named eight days following birth, during circumcision in a ceremony called a *bris* or *brit milah*. The ceremony for girls is called *brit bat* or *simchat bat* (celebration of the daughter) and usually takes place during regular Shabbat worship on the first Sabbath day after birth. In both instances scriptures are quoted, food is shared, and hopes for the child's future are toasted amongst friends and loved ones. In some Jewish homes, trees are planted at a child's birth. These trees will be cut down to form wood for the bridal canopy when the child is married.

Among certain Australian Aboriginal tribes, naming happens at birth. Names of relatives are recited while the baby is being born. The one spoken at the moment of birth is the name chosen for the child. The child will also have an inexorable bond with that relative for life. In Japan a boy is not given a public name until puberty, while in some Native American traditions a wide range of names is given across one's life: some for achievements, some for spiritual advancement, and some as clan names. Friends and relatives know certain names, and strangers know others. The name you are called by is based on who is doing the calling and what juncture you have reached in life.

Irish tradition was very specific about who had to be named after whom:

- first son after father's father
- second son after mother's father
- third son after father
- fourth son after father's oldest brother
- fifth son after mother's oldest brother
- first daughter after mother's mother (or father's mother)
- second daughter after father's mother (or mother's mother)
- third daughter after mother
- fourth daughter after mother's oldest sister
- fifth daughter after father's oldest sister

In many cultures, the baby's name serves as a connection between culture and the individual—between living people and the spirit world of ancestors. Some expectant mothers have had the unusual experience of having their baby give its own name in dreams or through intuition. "You should call me Benjamin, after your grandfather," a mother will dream, seeing the face of her unborn baby boy in front of her, or "I want to be named Linda, after your grandmother." Some believe that the baby may have a sense of purpose and use the name that will best suit them on their own heroic life journey.

In some African traditions, divination is used to determine the baby's proper name. By consulting with the ancestors and the spirit world, expectant parents can determine the spiritual identity of their unborn child and their corresponding name. This name will often express the child's purpose for incarnating and their mission, serving as a constant reminder of why they came here.

With these global rituals in mind, the process of naming your baby will hopefully seem less daunting. It is exciting to discover the perfect baby name.

Journeywork
Choosing the Right Name

Open your mind to clues that may be all around you. Call upon your ancestors, a close loved one who has passed on, or a wise family member whom you trust. Meditate and let your mind become receptive to guidance from the baby and the spirit world. Explore your own cultural heritage and discover its naming traditions. Consider the attributes and opportunities you'd like for your child, and search for a name that represents them.

Naming your baby is the start of seeing them as a full and separate person. But don't be discouraged if you find that you can't decide on a name before the baby is born. Many parents find that upon seeing their baby for the first time, they instantly know the right name. Some even feel compelled to abandon the name they had previously chosen in favor of something that comes to mind while looking into their baby's eyes just after birth. The spirit can be powerful and unpredictable, and it's important to create a space for magic as your mystical journey unfolds into motherhood. The right name will vibrate with the spiritual essence of your baby, and you will know it when you speak it.

 ·

Journaling Cue: Keep a list of the names you like and allow it to be fluid so you can add and remove names whenever you want.

Musical Magic

A number of studies have demonstrated that babies in utero show a significant response to musical stimulation.[32] Abrams et al. showed that by twenty-six weeks a baby's ears are developed. In this study, the babies' changing heart rates showed their response to various sounds. A small study with sixteen pregnant women showed that newborn babies who were exposed to musical stimulation in utero demonstrated increased imitation of sounds made by adults and appeared to have structured vocalization earlier than the infants who did not have musical stimulation in utero.

In an attempt to determine the effects of daily stimulation of music in utero, babies were exposed at thirty-two and thirty-eight weeks to ten minutes of music. In the study, there was a ten-minute control period with no music followed by a period of music with headphones on the mother's abdomen (the baby could hear the sound but the mother could not). In addition to white noise, three types of music were played: piano solo, choral, and rock. The mothers were asked to record the number and types of movements that their babies were making.

At six weeks old, the babies were monitored for:

- number of movements
- opening of eyes
- frowning and anxiety
- whether the baby was listening
- no response
- crying

At the thirty-two-week mark, the fetuses did not seem to differentiate between the types of music played. At thirty-eight weeks, there was an increased response to the choral and piano solo. And at six weeks after birth (postpartum), the babies who had been exposed to music in utero were more attentive, alert, and active.

Another study demonstrated that babies exposed to about seventy-two hours of music from the twenty-eighth week of pregnancy through birth demonstrated superiority in gross and fine motor development, verbal development, and some aspects of body control compared with the control group that was not exposed to music.

Dancing for Childbirth

Toward the conclusion of your pregnancy, your Braxton Hicks contractions are likely to occur more frequently and may be more intense. Some women describe these as similar to pain before or during a period. Coming, as they do, so close to labor, they represent the challenges a hero must undergo at the crowning of the journey. This is your opportunity to demonstrate that you have honed your abilities, strengthened your resolve, and prepared for the great test of your might. You have nearly reached the pinnacle of your journey, and you must be ready to surmount the ultimate challenge. When you view these contractions as preparation, you will hear Mother Nature whispering, "You can do it; you can birth your baby."

Contractions are kick-started by the hormone oxytocin, a powerful chemical that is also released during orgasm. Commonly known as "the love hormone," oxytocin facilitates physical and emotional bonding between lovers as well as between mother and child. Alternative birth practitioners describe mindful childbirth as "orgasmic" birth because it allows you to bring awareness to and intensify the positive effects of oxytocin. Your awareness of the spiritual presence in nature may grow stronger as you realize that your body has been equipped with this hormone, which not only stimulates contractions but also induces calm and bonds you to those you love. Rather than fearing the Braxton Hicks contractions, take advantage of the oxytocin that helps you become calmer and more comfortable in childbirth. Embrace the complex feelings that your body, in its wisdom, is offering you in advance of birth to prepare you for the peak of your pregnancy journey.

One of the ways to naturally release oxytocin and smooth the path to childbirth is through dancing and rhythmic movement. For centuries, Middle Eastern women have used traditional dance forms to mimic birth contractions and prepare their bodies for that big moment. Experiencing contractions prior to birth reduces fear and anxiety and teaches you what to expect. Over twenty years ago, a famous belly dancer named Morocco wrote about the connections between childbirth and this ancient art form:

> Oriental dancing, as the Arabs themselves call it, is one of the oldest forms of dance, originating with pre-biblical religious rites worshiping motherhood, and two of its movements (the only two actually done with the abdominal muscles) have as their practical side the preparation of females for the stresses of childbirth. Thus it is also, in a way, the oldest form of natural childbirth instruction.[33]

Morocco interviewed legendary dancers in Egypt, Morocco, and other countries where the tradition remained. What these women told her was that they performed the ancient dance as instruction for pregnant women, to train them to ride the contractions like waves. The waves are said to be taken from nature: from the movement of waves of the ocean (the mother of us all) and from the sinuous undulation of snakes when they are shedding their skins. (In the very ancient world, snakes and birth goddesses were worshiped together. In Aboriginal culture, the rainbow snake is the mother of creation.) Dance historian and woman's culture expert Wendy Buonaventura says:

> Dancing is…the expression…of a woman's entire life experience, whether it is used as a symbol of luck and fertility, an aid to childbirth, a means of passing the time, a form of therapy…The Arab idea of female beauty does not confine itself to the young and slim, but also takes in the quality of the voluptuous, with its hint of an enveloping protectiveness and sensual ease.[34]

The practice of women dancing for women was also common in the Turkish harems of the sultan in Istanbul's Topkapi palace. A visit to the palace reveals the private rooms where women danced for each other in anticipation of the ultimate goal—childbirth and a son for the sultan. Even today, women in Turkey often dance for each other at weddings or baby showers, encouraging and exclaiming over beautifully executed moves or particularly graceful "contractions."

While some exercise routines are difficult and dangerous during the last trimester of pregnancy, the gentle undulations of belly dancing can be modified and used to relax the pelvis and to gently rock your baby in the womb to the soothing sounds of music. You can also use these gentle moves not only to help ease the onset of Braxton Hicks contractions but to learn to release oxytocin and use its calming effects. Yogic breathing is a wonderful complement to these moves.

For women (and men), the rolling movements of belly dancing are also traditionally perceived as highly erotic. The erotic element has been romanticized from Victorian times to today and has diminished the dance's earliest beginnings as an aid and instruction for childbirth. Not only can you benefit from both the erotic and the practical uses of dance, you can also let it awaken your spirit. As you move rhythmically, gently releasing oxytocin into your system, you learn that the sensation of contractions brings forth a transcendent bond of love between you and your baby.

Journeywork
Dancing with Baby

Start with a calming and hypnotic piece of music that will last for at least twenty minutes at a slow pace.

Now light a natural candle or incense and turn off your cell phone. Put on some clothing that's light, pretty, and easy to move within (silk or something soft on your skin is optimum).

Stand with your weight evenly distributed between both legs. Raise your arms to your sides and let your hips slide out from underneath you. Roll them around to the left, then to the right. As you do so, raise your diaphragm upwards—notice your breathing easing as your ribcage gains space from the encroaching uterus pushing up on it. Feel the stretch on your tailbone and your lower back as the movement relaxes muscles tightened from holding the weight of your baby within.

Now put your hands on your belly and move your hips gently from side to side, keeping time with the music and caressing the skin on your abdomen. You're dancing with your baby. Right now your child can feel the gentle pressure of the womb holding them tight in an inner cuddle that keeps them in happy stasis until birth. Imagine also that your baby is smiling—a natural state for a third-trimester baby in the womb. They can also feel the movement of the amniotic fluid rocking softly as your hips move back and forth. They can hear the soft sounds of the music as you move. As you relax and feel pleasure, your baby absorbs the pleasure chemicals in your brain, which pass to them through your bloodstream.

Consider doing this traditional dance for your partner—a healthy way to initiate gentle sexuality and heightened sensuousness in the third trimester. Remember that the most powerful way to release oxytocin is through touch. Try inviting your partner to touch you softly as you move, and notice the sensations of pleasure, the connection between you, and the bond created between you, your partner, and your baby in this rhythm of life.

Spiritual Sensuality

The full blossoming of your pregnancy can be an incredibly erotic time. The increased blood and the pressure of your baby toward the birth canal can send extra sensation and lubrication to your vagina. As long as you practice the safety precautions your medical team has set out for you, you can look forward to pleasing sensations along with the life-affirming changes that motherhood brings. Most doctors agree that you can enjoy sexual bonding right up until you go into labor unless you're having a high-risk pregnancy.

Of course, whether or not you feel like making love is another question entirely. But on those days or evenings when you're feeling amorous, it's a good idea to allow yourself to go with the flow. Having an orgasm is one of the best ways for you and your partner to release tension and fall into a deep sleep. And the hormones that you both create through lovemaking engender a greater sense of security and courage in both of you and in the baby. Some doctors recommend having sex throughout the third trimester to smooth the way for delivery. Just avoid the woman on top position because all of the ligaments in your pelvic area are stretching and your cartridge is softening in preparation for birthing. The important thing to remember is that it's just as okay to pass on sex as it is to have it. And during this stage of your journey, skin-to-skin spooning can be just as soothing and bonding as making love.

As your journey crowns and you close the distance between pregnancy and birthing, your emotional state might best be described as bittersweet. You've been carrying this baby for almost nine months, and you're ready to meet them. But you're probably also feeling some melancholy or sadness about the physical separation that is imminent. Don't fixate on this state of mind. Invest your energy in your spiritual cleansing and nesting. Share music with the baby, and continue to dance together. As you do these things, your anticipation will grow, and by the time you go into labor, you will be ready to welcome your baby to the "outer world."

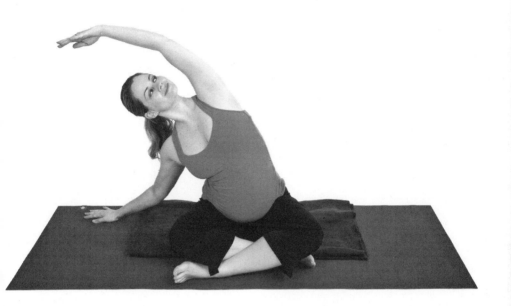

Yoga Pose
Side Stretch
Opening Both Sides of the Body

From a seated position on a folded blanket, place one hand down next to your body. Reach the other hand up and over your head, reaching toward your opposite side. Then repeat with the other hand. Each side of your body holds different energies and tensions. Pay attention to the subtle differences each side hold.

Benefits
- This pose stretches and lengthens one side of the body at a time, helping to create space and increase lung capacity, making breathing easier and maintaining spinal and muscular suppleness.

Precaution

As your pregnancy progresses, be sure you are grounded so that you don't lose your balance. Only stretch as far to one side or the other as feels comfortable.

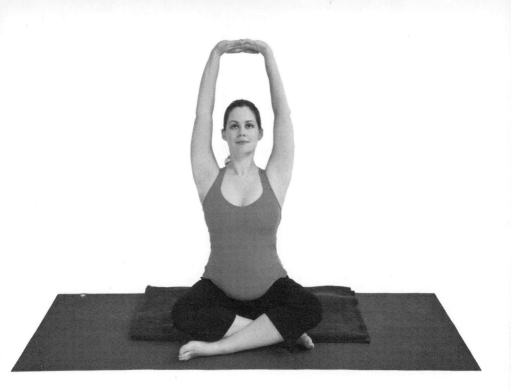

Yoga Pose
Opening the Heart
Strengthening the Bond

This yoga pose will help you to strengthen the heart-to-heart bond you already have with your baby.

Sit on the floor with your legs crossed or stretched out in front of you, in a chair or on your bed—whatever feels most comfortable.

Close your eyes. Balance your breathing by inhaling for eight seconds and exhaling for eight seconds. Maintain this pattern of breathing as you imagine you can see the roots of energy that connect your feet and the base of your spine with the earth. With each breath, feel this energy calming you and giving you strength.

Now slowly reach out with your hands until both arms are extended in front of you, parallel with the floor.

Clasp your hands together and slowly raise your hands above your head as you continue taking full, energizing breaths.

Take several full breaths with your hands overhead, and then gently lower your hands back down to your sides.

By reaching over your head, you're lengthening your spine and increasing the space between the bottom of your rib cage and your hip bones. As baby grows and takes up more space in your belly, this pose will help you to breathe more deeply.

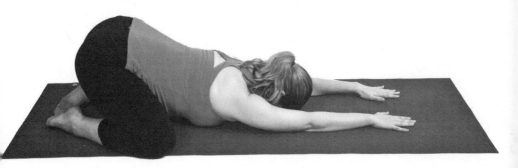

Yoga Pose
Child's Pose
Relaxation

Starting on your hands and knees, with your knees wide apart, sit back on your heels and stretch your arms out in front of you, placing your forehead on the floor. (Late in the third trimester, you can place a pillow under your head.)

Benefits

- Child's Pose can be a good resting and pelvic opening pose between contractions, alternating with Cat Pose.

- The center of the forehead has a pressure point that induces relaxation.

Precaution

This may not feel good during labor because it puts pressure on the perineum.

As you complete your third trimester, no longer is your identity solely about you; your baby is now becoming a part of who you are—a separate person who is nevertheless eternally connected through the sacred bond of mother and child. Your inner sense of divinity is growing as you meet the challenge of reimagining yourself. Even as your body shifts and changes, you are becoming more aware of and inspired by working together with your higher power to bring forth new life.

Part 4
Birth

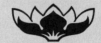

Behold the Holy Grail

Your baby enters the light of the world from the sacred space of the womb—dark, warm, protective, and nurturing waters. As a baby crosses that threshold and takes the first breath, we all marvel at the miracle of life. And as your newborn emerges, so do new sacred spaces in your life—concentric circles formed by parents and child, then spiraling out to encompass siblings, grandparents, aunts and uncles, cousins and friends. There is a new spirit in the world. A new chapter in the circle of life begins.

In all world cultures, ancient and modern, the miracle of birth is accompanied by ritualistic practices. Ancient Greeks removed all knotted materials from the birthing room and cleansed the baby right after birth to protect against bad luck. In ancient China, foul language was prohibited for fear of cursing the newborn, and babies were not cleansed for three days in order to strengthen them against evil influence. In Kenya, the father sits or stands outside the labor hut and takes the belt off his trousers to ritualistically release all constrictions so his wife and baby can have an easier birth.

As you prepare for the birth of your child, honor yourself by choosing the rituals that you believe will give you and the baby the most support, comfort, and peace of mind. We want you to look back on your birth experience with pride at what you've accomplished and awe for the miracle of life. We want you to be empowered by trusting your spiritual path and making time and space for the rituals that are most important to you. And while there are different beliefs and approaches for childbirth, in every case the intention is to bring a healthy new life into the world.

Chapter 7

Birth as Spiritual Awakening

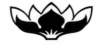

*When a baby is born, the mother
in particular enters into a new,
larger relationship with the world.*
Gavin de Becker,
Protecting the Gift

"Now that I know I can do it and what to expect, I'm excited about home birthing," said Ana, a vibrant twenty-eight-year-old with a three-year-old daughter. Ana's first experience giving birth was in a hospital, and it had gone smoothly. She said, "It was in a birthing suite, and I loved it. I'm not knocking hospital birthing; I just want to try it at home this time."

Monica, a forty-one-year-old mother of home-birthed twins, decided that her baby girl would be birthed in a hospital. "I loved giving birth to Ben and Amelia at home, but that was eight years ago. I know women my age and older home birth, but I think I'll feel more relaxed in a birthing suite at the hospital, just in case I need the extra support."

When it comes to giving birth, what's right for one woman may be wrong for another. We encourage our patients to learn about all their options and choose the place and method they feel good about. From birthing tents to high-tech hospitals, women can have babies where they desire (and sometimes where they don't). There is a movement toward delivering babies at home in the comfort of familiar surroundings, and celebrities Meryl Streep, Ricki Lake, and Nellie Furtado are part of that movement, along with Demi Moore, who did it three times. This movement back to natural childbirth was just getting started back in the 1980s when comedian Joan Rivers joked, "My idea of natural childbirth is wearing absolutely no makeup."

Jokes aside, birthing at home can be a wonderful experience for women who are healthy, have no known risks for safe delivery, and feel comfortable with this choice. But we don't want women who feel more comfortable in a hospital setting to think they're missing out. Women birthing at home should not be criticized, and neither should women choosing a hospital birth. Each experience is steeped in rituals, and this chapter will show you the rituals involved even in the depths of the surgical suite.

What we want you to focus on is that on your hero's journey, the new life you bring forth is your Holy Grail. This moment is what you have been working toward for the past nine months. As the birth canal opens you physically, your heart chakra will be opening you spiritually. Know that you are ready. You have risen above challenges, been tested by circumstances, withstood physical and emotional pain, and gained wisdom. Breathe easy and know that you are ready to receive your Holy Grail—your baby, body, mind, and spirit. As part of the rite of passage, you are tapping into the female energy of the world and all of the mothers who have gone before you. You are also tapping into the maternal energy of Mother Earth.

Journeywork
Honoring the Earth Mother

To draw on the grounding and nourishing aspects of Mother Earth, walk outside and face north. If it's warm, stand on the earth with your bare feet and feel the earth's heat as you ground yourself. If it's cold, imagine you can feel this heat. Then take a few deep breaths and imagine your feet growing roots. They extend down into the ground and spread out beneath you, firmly anchoring your energy to the earth. Say a prayer thanking the earth for giving and sustaining life. Thank her for being your home and for providing the water, minerals, and food that you and your baby need to live.

Leave an offering for the earth. It can be water, a strand of your hair, or a sprinkling of tobacco. Now turn to your right and slowly walk in small, ever-widening circles until you see a stone or pebble that calls to you. Perhaps it shines or looks smooth. Maybe it has a design or shape that appeals to you. You cannot choose incorrectly. Select the stone you like, hold it close to your belly, and tell the baby that you are both part of the earth and this stone represents this connection. Take a moment to say a prayer—perhaps the following Navajo birth blessing or one of your own favorites.

"From the heart of Earth by means of yellow pollen, blessing is extended. Blessing is extended. On top of a pollen floor may I there in blessing give birth! With long life-happiness surrounding me, may I in blessing give birth! May I quickly give birth. In blessing may I arise again. In blessing may I recover. As one who is long life-happiness, may I live on!"

Bring the stone home and place it on your birthing altar or in a safe place in the nursery.

Transitioning Through the Pain

Whether you birth in the hospital or at home, pain is part of the journey. Fortunately, your body is designed to help you to feel more comfortable through it all. Dimethyltryptamine is a naturally occurring hallucinogen that is released when you're stressed. Birth is a naturally stressful process for you and the baby, so it's not a far leap to assume that DMT is being released simultaneously within you and your baby. As you transition from the first stage of labor into a more active stage and begin pushing, DMT is likely helping you along. We've often noticed that when women who have not received pain medication are 7–8 centimeters dilated, they appear to be having an out-of-body experience. It's almost as if they don't feel the intensity of the pain. At this stage, many women have their eyes closed, as if they are in deep meditation or trance. Later, these women typically say they don't remember much about that phase of their labor.

Our theory is that this is the time when DMT is being released into the bloodstream from the maternal pineal gland. This release of DMT provides greatly needed pain relief. If the mother and baby are releasing DMT simultaneously, this could be the ultimate spiritual point where bonding occurs. The accounts of indigenous shamans who use plant medicines that contain substances like DMT in rituals often include out-of-body journeys. Some say they travel to the center of the world, called the axis mundi—the point where heaven and hell connect. The axis mundi has also been described as an umbilical cord attached to the perceived world, providing spiritual nourishment. During this phase of labor, do mothers spiritually travel to the axis mundi to connect with their soon-to-be-born babies? We can't prove it, but we believe the answer is yes.

So what about women who receive epidurals? Do they forfeit the chance to experience this axis mundi communion with their babies? Not necessarily. Even without intense pain, birthing is stressful, so it's likely that some DMT is being released for these women and their babies too. But beyond the question of the help from DMT, we believe that by bonding with your baby during the months leading up to birth, the communication channel is already established, so mother and baby can spiritually meet at the axis mundi or anywhere else. But the axis mundi is a very appropriate meeting place when you consider that it is at the center of the world and baby is at the center of you.

Journeywork
Aromatherapy for Birthing

A study conducted in a maternity ward in the United Kingdom indicates that aromatherapy in the birthing room is effective in normalizing childbirth. They also reported an increase in maternal satisfaction with the labor experience. Of note, staff members who were interviewed also demonstrated a desire to continue providing the aromatherapy service because they believed it positively affected the labor and birth.

Select a couple aromatherapy oils to take with you to the hospital or have nearby if you're birthing at home. Citrus and peppermint are great to increase alertness, while lavender and oats can help you to relax.

Home Birth as a Rite of Passage

Late one afternoon as Carly was washing dishes, her water broke. With her labor beginning, she texted her husband. He forwarded the message to her sister and mother, who were both invited to participate in the home birth. Everything in her birthing room had been ready for more than a week, so she decided to relax and soak in a warm bath. She'd stashed her favorite salted caramels in the bathroom for this very moment, and she savored one as she talked to the baby, telling him that they were a team and that together this transition would be a beautiful spiritual event and a bonding experience for both of them and Daddy too.

For Carly, the bath wasn't just soothing, it was also part of her birthing ritual. Like centuries of women before her, she was immersing herself in clear water not only to cleanse her body but also to spiritually prepare herself for the miracle of birth. Other rituals would follow this one, but for now Carly was focused only on her breathing and connecting with her baby. She had decided to birth on her living room floor this time but wondered about trying water birthing next time.

In her paper "Reinscribing the Birthing Body: Home Birth as Ritual Performance," Melissa Cheyney, a medical anthropologist and licensed midwife, eloquently describes the ritual phases of home birth. She divides the experience into the three phases of separation, transition, and reintegration. The separation phase covers prenatal care, the transition phase is labor and childbirth, and the reintegration phase takes place after the baby is born.[35] Cheyney interviewed mothers and midwives to learn about their home-birthing process and look for common threads and approaches. From these, she developed the following stages:

The Separation Phase

This is the first phase and begins when you discover you're pregnant. Excitement, joy, and sometimes a little fear or apprehension characterize this prenatal phase. Ritualistically, many women usher in this phase with a new look at diet and exercise, realizing that everything they eat, drink, and do may affect their unborn child. Cheyney believes that women who choose give birth at home may enjoy this phase of pregnancy more than those who choose hospital birth because they are investing less in labs and ultrasounds and also have less apprehension in terms of waiting for the results. Home birth is a choice to separate from technology where women enter a trusting relationship with a midwife who is grounded in her years of experience and her intimate understanding of being female. But from our experience, women who are choosing hospital births can enjoy this phase just as much, providing they stay calm and centered by using our yoga poses and journeywork.

The mechanization of medicine has fostered the concept that the female body can't have a safe birth without intervention. This concept makes many women worry that home birthing may be an unnecessary risk. Of course, the women who do it successfully see this very differently, and a midwife can help strengthen your conviction once your decision to give birth at home is made. One of the most powerful gifts the midwife offers is her understanding that your body was made to give birth. The body that has conceived, nourished, and protected your unborn baby doesn't become faulty when it's time to deliver; it continues to know exactly what to do and is structured perfectly to deliver your child.

When you acknowledge this truth, you're not only standing up to the modern paradigm, you're also engaging your feminine power. This opens your heart and mind to the wisdom of your body. During the months leading up to your baby's birth, the midwife acts as officiator and visits you in your home, taking the time to connect with you and get to know you, your desires, and any fears you might have. The beauty of this is that you undergo your prenatal care in the same facility where you'll deliver your baby. You eat, sleep, play, entertain, meditate, and daydream there, and soon you will deliver your baby there too.

> **Journaling Cue:** Write yourself an affirmation that reflects your belief and trust in your body's wisdom, such as: "My body knows what to do. Women have been having babies for thousands of years, and I will trust in my body's wisdom and in the strength of the women giving birth before me."

This strong sense of home is conveyed to the baby throughout the prenatal phase, which is meant to strengthen the bond between you, the baby, and the midwife. Your midwife will also encourage the use of tests and diagnostic procedures, and she will take the time to explain why the tests can be helpful. She will also help you to understand the test results and use this knowledge as power.

One of the most meaningful aspects of birthing at home is having your loved ones with you during delivery, instead of outside in a waiting room. Whether it's just you, your partner, and the midwife or you're surrounded by your other children, extended family members, and close friends, the baby is entering the world in the presence of their new family. Symbolically and literally, this practice acknowledges that it takes a village to raise a child. It also hearkens back to indigenous cultures where women often birth in front of their children and the birthing process is considered a natural part of life where women are in charge. Some women ask their loved ones to dress in celebratory clothing, as if they are going to a party, while others may request that everyone wear white or her favorite color. One of our patients wanted everyone in the room to wear a different color so the entire spectrum of the rainbow would be in the birthing room with her. And some women want everyone to wear whatever they feel most comfortable in, whether that's jeans and T-shirt, flannel pajamas, or a tailored suit. What's important is that you put yourself and the baby first in making these choices. No one's opinions are important as your own at this time.

As you look upon your home as the sacred space for delivery, you're also looking upon your body as a sacred space for the baby. In your epic journey, you are the vessel carrying the sacred Holy Grail. Having this understanding makes it easier to be gentle with yourself, eat healthy food, drink clean water, breathe fresh air, and exercise.

It's a good idea to decide where in your home you want to give birth at least a few weeks before your due date. Together with the baby's father, you can consecrate this space by creating an altar that is adorned with items that symbolize your love for each other and your shared joy for the new life you will soon bring into the world. If you have children, they can participate in this ritual too. They may choose to draw a picture to put on the altar or to put one of their favorite toys, dolls, or action figures on the altar to show their support for the changes you're all going to experience with the addition of a new member of the family. You can set an intention with objects or prayers you place on the altar and gain strength from these offerings once your labor begins. Once the room is cleansed and the altar is made, you will be in the perfect spiritual space to decide who you want to be with you during labor and delivery. Keep in mind that you can ask people to be with you in spirit who aren't able to travel to the birthing location. The sacred power of divine spirit transcends space and time.

By the time birth is ready to begin, your home will have been transforming over nine months, not just physically but energetically. Preparations will have been made to create space not only for baby to grow and thrive after birth but to enter this world—a magical portal through which the unborn becomes born. Standard hospital equipment is replaced by objects that support the natural progression of birth. IV poles are replaced with coat racks, fetal monitors replaced with speakers for music, and instead of withholding food, you're welcome to enjoy any nourishing foods or beverages that you desire. Cheyney describes the high-touch aspects of home birth as opposed to the high-tech aspects of hospital birth and how the physiologic aspects of touch take women into a luminal phase she calls "laborland."

The endpoint of this phase for home birth is the clear understanding that it is women—not doctors or hospitals—who produce babies. That said, we encourage women who opt for natural home births to have an ob-gyn they trust on their birthing team as backup. Should something occur that can't be easily handled at home, the doctor can meet you at the hospital and already have all the necessary information. When we play this backup role, we set the intention that our assistance will not be needed, but when something unexpected happens and we *are* needed, we're relieved that we can help. In most cases, our main role during labor and delivery is to offer support from afar by holding the mother and baby in our consciousness and envisioning them enveloped in divine light.

The Transition Phase

When the baby moves into the lower region of your womb, you'll know that birthing is soon to follow. This is a good time to physically and energetically cleanse the birthing room. Some women enjoy doing this alone as part of their nesting rituals, while other women prefer to include other people in this process. To energetically cleanse the room, you can sing, chant, drum, clap, burn sage or sweetgrass, laugh, play harmonious music, or do a combination of all of these. Create a cleansing practice and ritual that feels good to you and makes you happy and calm.

Once labor begins, you will want to cleanse yourself and the other participants. In addition to the ritualistic cleansing, your participating loved ones may choose to bring gifts to place on the altar. These are not baby gifts so much as offerings that reflect their love for you or symbolize support. In the story of the birth of Jesus, the gifts given to Mary were gold, frankincense, and myrrh. These gifts were often given to kings, but frankincense and myrrh were also used for anointing, and gold symbolized extreme value. Scholars have speculated that myrrh and frankincense may have been given as antiseptic herbs for help with the birth. If you're a Christian or you simply like the symbolism, you might request that these gifts be among the ones you are given. But the offerings your loved ones bring can be much more affordable than gold! And for many mothers, the most valuable gifts are often the least expensive but most meaningful, including the homemade ones.

As your labor progresses, your midwife will encourage you to do whatever your body wants you to do. As with pregnancy itself, women around the world tend to follow the wisdom of their female ancestors. Some women laboring in Sudan scream throughout the birthing process to ward off the "evil eye," while women in this country sometimes think more quiet birth is better for the baby. These are decisions that are yours to make, so choose whatever is most empowering for you.

Intermittently, she will hook up a fetal monitor to check in on the baby's heart rate. A standard practice is to monitor the heart rate every fifteen minutes or so until you begin pushing, then every five minutes after that. In a home birth, no one will tell you to lie flat on your back or when to push. When Shawn was a young resident in a pregnancy ward, he was a disciplined acolyte of the hospital birthing process and thought the right way for women to give birth was to follow the standard birthing protocol of pushing during contractions.

One day as he was encouraging a young woman to keep pushing, she turned to him and said, "I'm not pushing anymore." He was speechless, since up to that point he had thought she *had* to keep pushing for the baby to be born. But her certainty in that moment was greater than his own, so he intuitively felt that she knew what she had to do better than he did. Not sure what else to do, he handed her the nurse call button and told her to push the button when she was ready to have the baby. About forty minutes later, the light came on, and when he arrived in her room, she said, "I'm ready." She pushed twice and the baby was born.

As Shawn tells it, "There is nothing that anyone could have said to prepare me for what happened that day. And while I still valued my medical training, I was in awe of the body wisdom and spiritual fortitude that allowed this woman to give birth, virtually with no help from me, except to catch the baby as it entered the world."

The Reintegration Phase

This phase begins once the baby is born and continues for weeks or months to come. When your baby emerges, your midwife will place it carefully on your belly without clamping or cutting the umbilical cord. Mother and baby are given some time to establish their new connection outside the womb while still being physically connected as they were before baby was born. As your new baby rests on your belly, you can touch them for the very first time. You can see the fingers and toes you've been envisioning in your journeywork and dreams and officially welcome them into the world. Once the cord stops pulsating, the midwife or father (or whomever you choose) can clamp and cut it.

Journeywork
Watching the Miracle Unfold

Place a hand mirror in your birthing room. As your cervix dilates, take a moment to look at the amazing transformation that your body is making. Each time you look at the progress you're making, allow the physical image of what you see to rest in your mind's eye. Set the mirror down, close your eyes, and visualize your vaginal opening as the gateway to this world. With your inner eyes, see your baby preparing for his or her grand entrance.

Hospital Birth as a Rite of Passage

Giant snowflakes rained down on Beth and JT as they made their way through the spring blizzard to the car. Fortunately, the storm crews had been out all day, so the roads were mostly clear on the way to the hospital. Before leaving home, Beth had changed into a warm pair of leggings, her Ugg boots, and one of her favorite pregnancy T-shirts—blue, hand-dyed, and super soft. She said, "The T-shirt made my belly look like the earth. Once we got there and I settled into my birthing room, I changed into my swimsuit and labored in the heated bathtub. That was very nice."

After the warm bath, rather than donning a hospital-issue robe, Beth got back into her T-shirt and leggings and kept the leggings on until she received her epidural. She kept her comfy "Mama Earth" shirt on during delivery and drew strength from the visual reminder that she was about to give earth a new child. She said she felt calm, safe, and enveloped in the divine essence of love.

Beth's story is one of millions illustrating that there's no right or wrong place to give birth. If you feel more comfortable or safer with the idea of a hospital birth, you can make it just as meaningful and ritualistic as a home birth. More than 90 percent of deliveries occur inside a hospital, and when you examine what happens in that setting, you'll see that rituals abound. The challenge is that these rituals are performed out of protocol rather than being directed by you. The key is to take charge of your labor and delivery plan and be sure you have an ob-gyn who supports your choices. The more you understand the hospital protocol for labor and delivery, the more you can align your spiritual intent with those practices. When the nurse comes in to check your blood pressure, rather than thinking of it as an intrusion, you can embrace it as a time to calm and center yourself and connect spiritually to the baby.

When we look at a hospital birth through the lens of ritual and spiritual involvement, even the mundane becomes a step in your journey toward delivery. By honoring your intention to receive your Holy Grail in the most spiritually joyful way, you can transcend the limitations of the physical world and intuitively guide the baby into this new world. The breathing and meditation exercises we shared throughout the book will help you to stay grounded and centered. We suggest recording or photocopying your favorites and bringing them along when you go into labor.

Birthing your baby is a rite of passage. While it is part of your hero's journey, it is also a journey within itself. On a journey within a journey, you will be walking with one foot in the spirit world and one foot in the physical. As your labor progresses, you will cover the same territory that you traveled on your nine-month journey to this event. The first pangs of labor are your call to adventure. You hesitate, not being sure, and then accept this call by phoning your partner and your doctor and gathering your pre-packed hospital bags. Getting from your house to the hospital is such an epic part of this journey that it's made it into numerous films—from dramas to comedies. In the excitement, it's not unusual to forget something, with the classic example being the husband rushing out the door without his wife.

This is the "ordeal" part of the journey, and keeping a sense of humor will allow it to be a comedy of errors instead of a series of unfortunate events.

When Katie went into labor with our first child, we were five weeks premature. When we arrived at the hospital, the baby was breech and having minor distress. The decision for cesarean section was made, and Shawn ran out to the car to get the camera that we forgot to bring in. By the time he got back, Katie was already in the OR with the spinal in place. Shawn almost didn't make the delivery! Thankfully, everything went well—and we remembered to bring the camera when our next three kids were born.

Your arrival at the hospital is representative of reaching the place in the inmost cave where your treasure awaits you. Now is the time for you, as the hero, to claim that treasure, and sometimes that means fighting for it. You have learned a great deal during the past nine months, and these last hours are your final test and trial. Sink into yourself, breathe deeply, and connect with your spiritual essence and that of your baby's as you move through the hospital rituals that will support your delivery.

When you arrive at the hospital and check in, you will be crossing the threshold from the "ordinary world" to the unfamiliar, even if this isn't your first birth. After you check in, you'll be given an identification bracelet. While not the most fashionable of accessories, this will be one of your first physical links to your baby after birth. Soon your baby will have a bracelet too, linking them to you. Once this is complete, you will most likely be met with an attendant and a wheelchair. This is for practical purposes as well as legal ones. Nobody wants a woman in labor to fall down during a contraction, so have a seat and enjoy the ride. You are the hero, remember, so it's only fitting that you be ushered through the next gateway with the help of others. You are the queen, and this is your throne on wheels.

Journeywork
Preparing for the Road Ahead

Prior to your delivery, ask family and friends to write messages of love and welcome to the baby and put them in sealed envelopes. You and your partner can do the same thing and have them in the room with you. Keep them close by the bed, drawing strength from the people in your life who could not be present but are with you in spirit. After your delivery, open the letters one by one and read them aloud, releasing the power of the stories and messages. These make lovely entries in your baby book too.

Energetically Cleansing Your Room or Suite

When you arrive in the room where you will complete your labor or the birthing suite where you will labor and deliver, you can energetically cleanse the room. Play some of your favorite music and spray a little of your favorite perfume or an essential essence like lime or lavender. Sit on the sofa or bed and center yourself.

Breathe deeply and slowly as you envision white, soothing light enveloping the baby and you and spreading out to fill the entire room. Set the intention that you will follow in the footsteps of all your female ancestors, and hold your connection to your spirit as well as your body as you complete this stage of your journey.

Bring your special stone from the journeywork exercise at the beginning of this chapter and place it in the room with you. You may also want to display a photo of your children or an illustration of a goddess who has given you strength during your journey. Placing just a few items around your room is a way of energetically claiming it and making it your own.

Journaling Cue: Now that the room is yours, take a few minutes to sit quietly and balance your breathing. Focus on everything and everyone you feel grateful for. Silently thank these people and offer gratitude for the events until you feel your heart start to open. You may even have some tears of gratitude. Ask your soul to give you a message for the hours ahead, and write this message down. If you are too keyed up to hear a message, write down what you believe your soul would share with you at this time.

Finding Your Pain Threshold

First of all, there is nothing wrong with wanting to experience childbirth with less pain. As with where to give birth, deciding whether you want the pain-reducing procedure called an epidural is entirely your call. You can also decide how much pain reliever you'd like. For instance, Sarah asked for a low-dose epidural. She said, "I wanted to be able to feel my contractions and when to push—and, more importantly, how hard to push. I had enough to take the pain edge off but could still feel a lot of pressure and bodily sensations that I would not describe as pain."

Some women know they want epidural before they even begin labor, and others want to wait and see if they want it after labor progresses for a while. Either of these routes is fine, but if you choose to wait, when you check in to the hospital be sure your anesthesiologist is aware of this. We've seen epidurals placed when women are completely dilated and we've seen anesthesiologists say they can't do it when a woman is dilated eight centimeters. So each case is different, but no matter how dilated you are, if the pain is so intense that you can't sit perfectly still for the procedure, the anesthesiologist won't be able to do it.

One of the arguments against epidurals is that they can slow labor, and there's some research that implies epidurals are a reason for the increased rates of cesarean section. But epidurals definitely assist many women who would otherwise have a much more challenging delivery. We encourage women to try laboring without medications until they reach a point where they feel incapable of proceeding without some relief. The epidural can allow you to relax and sleep. It can give you a chance to reflect and collect your thoughts on what you have accomplished up to this point.

Some women are surprised by how far they can go before asking for pain control, and others deliver naturally when they were not planning to do so. Recently, we've seen an increase in women choosing hypnotic birth instead of epidurals for pain control. This form of imagery and controlled breathing can bring about an epidural-like sense of pain control. With hypnosis there will be pain, but you can learn to harness it through breathing and controlled imagery.

Replacing Water and Minerals

In the not-too-distant past, it was standard practice to hook up an IV to women in labor to administer fluids intravenously and prevent her from becoming dehydrated. But in most hospitals today, you won't have an IV tube inserted as standard procedure if your birth plan says you don't want one. You can go through labor and birthing without an IV if you don't have epidural for pain and if you don't have any complications or physical symptoms that need the IV support.

If you have an epidural, IV fluids are routinely administered beforehand to reduce the chances of a drop in your blood pressure, which is a common side effect of this method of pain relief. Having the IV in place also makes it faster and easier for your doctor to administer any medications that you may need. If your doctor puts you on an IV, request a pole that has wheels. That will allow you walk around, change positions on the bed, and use any labor positions that feel good to you.

We often ask our patients to allow the IV without the fluid attached so we will have immediate access to the vein in the event of an emergency. Having the IV tube inserted without being attached to the hydration pouch gives you free range without dragging a pole around with you. Since Sarah put off her epidural until she was close to active labor, she was only hooked up to the IV and fetal heart monitor for a few hours.

Journeywork
Baby's Heartbeat

Some women say that hearing the fetal heart rate through the monitor is music to their ears and others say it increases their anxiety. We suggest that you spiritually align yourself with your baby's heartbeat to make this technology be a help rather than a hindrance. When you're laboring, breathe deeply and mindfully and listen to the baby's heartbeat. Listen as it increases and decreases in tempo. Imagine your own heart rate increasing as you inhale and decreasing as you exhale. With each inhalation, you fill your lungs with oxygen that traverses miles of blood vessels as it crosses the placental venous tree and fills your baby's bloodstream with oxygen. With each exhale, you're giving back to the universe what the baby has given to you. You can also rest easy knowing that the heart monitor will alert your doctor of any impending issues.

Your Birthing Positions

In most hospital deliveries today, laboring mothers are reclining on their backs, but this practice is shifting as women take back their intuitive power to birth as their own bodies dictate. We believe that you're the best person to decide the position in which you will give birth, but not all ob-gyns agree, so be sure to have this discussion with your doctor *before* you go into labor. Some women like being on their backs because they can push their feet into the stirrups, giving them more power to push. And if you've had an epidural, you'll have no option but to be on your back, because your legs won't have the power to support you in a squatting or standing position.

We've both delivered many babies with women who were in a squatting position. If you're strong enough, this can be a very productive position, as gravity helps pull the baby downward. In outdoor births, a small bowl-shaped area is dug up and lined with soft, clean materials so that the baby will have a soft landing position. The laboring mother squats over this "earth bowl," which is large enough to hold the baby once they are born. In a hospital setting, you will most likely be squatting on a birthing bed. Some women alternate between squatting and being on their hands and knees. This gives your leg and back muscles a break, and if you lower your buttocks to meet your heels, it can be a comfortable pushing and birthing position.

Draping and Prepping

Once doctors discovered that a clean environment was beneficial for the mother and the baby, it became commonplace to drape the laboring woman's legs with blue surgical drapes and prep the vulva and vagina with a bacteriostatic cleaning agent. Up until around the mid-1990s, standard procedures often included trimming pubic hair and administering an enema to empty the bowels prior to pushing the baby out. Today, things are typically quite different, with none of these preparatory steps being taken, because we realize they are unnecessary unless we need to perform a C-section. That said, if you would feel more comfortable with the added privacy of draping, feel free to request it.

To Cut or Not to Cut?

Up until the early twenty-first century, doctors believed that making a short, shallow incision between the vagina and rectum (the area called the perineum) would hasten the birthing process and prevent extensive tearing. They also believed that this straight incision would heal faster and better than the sorts of small tears that occur naturally during childbirth. While this seemed like a good idea at the time, we later learned that this procedure, called an episiotomy, is not always the best route to take. At that point, the standard changed, and we stopped doing routine episiotomies. Today, most doctors perform them only when they are truly needed. We consider this option if extensive vaginal tearing seems likely, if the baby is not in a headfirst position, or if the baby needs to be delivered quickly.

If your doctor feels this procedure will assist you, they will be sure that you do not feel any pain when the incision is made or when it's stitched after you give birth. If you haven't had an epidural or other anesthesia (or if it is starting to wear off), you will probably be given an injection that will numb the area. If this procedure becomes part of your hero's journey, use your conscious intention to focus on this being a necessary process to open your baby's first gateway to the world. Allow yourself to feel gratitude for the episiotomy, since it is helping baby to cross the threshold into their own life journey.

The Main Event

Once your active labor begins, we encourage you to stay tuned to your body's innate wisdom channel and give yourself permission to try whatever you're being guided to do. How does it feel when you push? Would pushing harder feel better or worse? Do you want to be warmer or cooler? Do you want sips of water or ice chips? You're the only one who will know the right answers to these questions. Trust yourself. And to the extent that you can, revel in these final hours of your spiritual pregnancy. Talk to the baby and let them know you and Daddy are waiting with open arms to embrace and love them. Feel the power of your life-giving contractions. Sit in awe of the spiritual being that you are about to greet in physical form. On this epic journey, you are the life-giving vessel, the carrier of the Holy Grail.

Prior to beginning active labor, be sure you let your doctor know how you want things to go once the baby is born. Will Daddy be the baby catcher or will he clamp and cut the cord?

Some hospitals' protocol might not coincide with your preferences, but there are usually compromises that can be made.

If you want to have the placenta saved so that you can plant it, cover this with your doctor ahead of time. Many hospitals have policies that make the placenta hospital property after it delivers. However, if you have religious or spiritual rituals regarding the tissues, many hospitals will waive these policies for you. Some mothers like to create a placental tree by planting a new tree with the placenta placed at its roots. This tree is an offering to the planet on behalf of your new baby. If you want to do this, have someone freeze the placenta for you so it will be preserved for your planting day.

Whether you take home the placenta or not, we encourage you to take a look at it. Notice its shape, size, and color. The placenta was attached to you and also to the sac your baby lived in for the past nine months. Your body grew this life-giving organ from the cells and tissues of your body so you could feed and protect your baby.

The Love Hormone

No matter where you give birth, you will be supported by your body in myriad ways that science still doesn't completely understand. One of the ways your body will rise to the occasion is through a hormone called oxytocin, often referred to as the love, or cuddle, hormone. Both you and the baby experience heightened levels of oxytocin at the time of birth. The word *oxytocin* itself comes from the Greek *kytokin* and means "quick birth." It's called the love hormone because it's stimulated in the mother during birth, helps to facilitate breastfeeding, and is also a bonding hormone, being released during intimate touch and orgasm.

During the birthing process, your brainwaves also begin processing information at deeper alpha levels, and finally at even deeper theta levels. This is sometimes called the "birth trance." Mothers report that this trance can be as ecstatic as sexual climax. Your oxytocin levels will continue to be elevated after birth and may be part of the emotional mother/child bonding experience. And your brain-wave changes continue after birth too, ushering in a heightened state of awareness.

Unexpected Twists and Turns

On a hero's journey, unexpected twists and turns are not uncommon, and this is true with your spiritual pregnancy journey as well. Sometimes the course of your birthing journey is altered by the position of the baby or the umbilical cord or by an unexpected turn of events. In these cases, your doctor may determine that the best choice for you and the baby is to surgically remove the baby through your abdominal wall instead of risking vaginal delivery. Doctors agree that this surgery, called a cesarean section or C-section, should be done only when necessary. But determining whether or not it's necessary is a bit of a tightrope walk. Our goal is to allow the labor and delivery to progress on its own unless we see signs that mean mother or baby may come to harm if we don't intervene. In the next chapter, we'll guide you through the possibility of an assisted delivery or a C-section and show you how these experiences can play important roles in your hero's journey.

Whether you choose to birth in a hospital with the aid of pain-reducing medication or you opt for natural birth at home, you will experience the miracle of your baby's first breath. To inspire literally means to inhale. Baby's first inspiration will fill her lungs with life-giving oxygen and fill your heart with immeasurable bliss whether you birth at home, in the hospital, or in the back seat of a cab. In that magical moment, all will be right in your world.

Chapter 8

Surgery as a Spiritual Ritual

*I'm beginning to perceive motherhood
as a long, slow letting go, of which
birth is just the first step.*
Sandra Steingraber, *Having Faith*

Stephanie, a twenty-eight-year-old artist and first-time mother-to-be, had everything planned for a natural childbirth in a birthing suite at the same hospital where she had been born. She and her husband, Tim, had taken a Lamaze breathing class and practiced yoga and meditation throughout the pregnancy. They were both excited to finally meet the baby boy that Stephanie was carrying. But she had proceeded to seven centimeters and had stayed there for over four hours with no cervical change, despite adequate contractions and the ability to rest. When we told Stephanie we needed to choose a different course of action, she burst into tears.

She said, "I didn't even want an epidural, and now I have to have surgery? What went wrong? Is my baby going to be okay? Am I?"

We were able to answer her questions and put her mind at ease, and after discussing it with us and with Tim, she decided to move forward with a C-section.

Even though we prepare our patients for this unlikely possibility, it's never easy for them to hear—and it's never easy for us to say either. But from our perspective, bringing a new life into the world is a miracle whether it happens naturally or with surgical assistance. And as we told Stephanie, "The first time you hold your baby and look into his eyes, the way he got here won't matter one bit."

We explained to Stephanie that with an epidural or a spinal block, she would be numb but she'd still be conscious. In emergencies, sometimes general anesthesia is used that does put the woman to sleep with a quiet mind, and some women feel it's easier to connect with their babies spiritually. We have heard stories of dreams women have had during general anesthesia C-sections where they're holding or cuddling their babies. Many of these women believe they were spiritually communing with their baby while they were unconscious, and we have no reason to believe otherwise.

Stephanie would be having an epidural and a spinal block, so she would be awake and be able to witness the birth. This made her happy, but she was still frightened. We encouraged her and Tim to breathe together and visualize a spiritual bridge between each other and between them and the baby. After they completed the breathing exercise, Tim put on classical music by Vivaldi, one of Stephanie's favorite composers, and she continued her slow, deep breathing while Tim spoke soothingly to her and the baby, assuring them that all would be well. Once she felt calm and centered again, we inserted an IV to provide fluids and give us a gateway to administer medications if we determined that we needed to do so.

If you receive the news that a C-section is needed, the sooner you surrender to the reality and open yourself to your connection with spirit, the more centered and calm you will be when it's time for surgery. While the stereotypical images that come to mind when you hear the words "operating room" may have a frightening, negative, or technological connotation for you, this area of the hospital, and of surgery itself, is steeped in ritual.

In fact, medical science evolved from religion and spirituality,[36] with spirituality being more focused on individual growth, less formal, less authoritarian and orthodox, and more universalizing.[37] To this day, both medicine and spirituality can play a part in the relief of suffering and ultimately healing. And while we do what we can to prevent or reduce the amount of suffering our patients experience, we are aware that physical and emotional pain is sometimes a powerful motivator of spiritual growth and awakening. In the event that you're told you need to have a C-section, we hope you will open yourself to this transformative potential.

For example, studies have shown that people undergoing coronary artery bypass surgery often gain a new appreciation for life and health, and spirituality develops as an inner strength, helping them navigate through suffering.[38] And when we consider that medicine has its roots in religion, spirituality, and ritual, then the operating room takes on a sacred essence and so does surgery itself. Like the inmost cave of the hero's journey, the operating room is a restricted area that not many people are permitted to enter. When you cross the threshold into the surgical suite, you surrender your body and conscious mind and sink into your unconsciousness, where the material world loses its hold on you and the veil to the spirit world is thin. And when you consider all of the aspects of surgery—from preparation through recovery— you see that surgery has all the components of a sacred ritual. And while chances are good that you won't travel to this inmost cave on your hero's journey, it is our hope that seeing this world through our eyes will help you to appreciate the beauty of the ritual.

 ·····················

Journaling Cue: Describe the birthing experience that you would like to have. Be as detailed as possible. Be sure to discuss your desires with your doctor well ahead of time.

The Ritual Begins with Informed Consent

When surgical intervention is needed, your doctor will explain what needs to be done and why. We encourage you to ask questions so you can understand what's going on and know why your doctor believes the surgery needs to be done. Once you have the information, if you choose to follow your doctor's medical advice, you need to give your informed consent before the surgery proceeds. Essentially, informed consent is a process of communicating between patient and physician resulting in an authorization or agreement to undergo a specific healing intervention.[39]

There is a power in healing ritual, such as surgery, and some have attributed this power to the act of placebo[40]; if the patient is aware the ritual is for them, they may heal simply through this knowledge. A recent study of patients undergoing a placebo-controlled arthroscopic surgery showed similar success rates to patients actually undergoing the surgical procedure.[41] This study shows the power of preoperative counseling, preparation for the ritual or procedure, and how the incision can have the power to heal even when nothing surgical is performed.

In our practice it's obvious that the time spent counseling our patients about the surgical process is the preparatory work of the ritual. One of the first things moms having C-sections want to know is whether their partner can be in the OR with them. We're pleased to let moms know that most anesthesiologists will allow one or two people to accompany them into the surgical suite.

Once we answer all the pressing questions, we give our preparatory instructions:

- no food or drink after midnight the night before
  (to make sure they have an empty stomach)
- bring an approved car seat for the baby, along with a
  couple changes of clothes for both mom and baby
- call our office with any questions
  so we can discuss them

This preparatory work is treated as sacred, and the C-section could be canceled if the directions are not followed exactly as prescribed. This process resembles certain spiritual practices such as those in the Brazilian church Uniao do Vegetal, which will not allow members to participate in the sacramental plant rituals if they do not follow strict diets and abstain from certain behaviors.[42]

If you're having a C-section, your doctor will provide you with a list of foods and drugs to avoid before surgery. We advise our patients to refrain from meats that are not fresh, deli meats, smoked and fermented food (including tofu and bean curd), aged cheeses, liquid or powder protein mixes, shrimp paste, sauerkraut, overripe fruits, aspartame, fava beans, caffeine, chocolate, raspberries, and peanuts. (If you groaned when you read chocolate, pack some in your bag for your recovery.) There are also many drugs to avoid like pseudoephedrine (Sudafed), Benadryl, antidepressants, and anti-nausea medicines, so check with your doctor before taking any drugs during this preparatory stage.

The process of preparation is what sets the tone for a sacred ritual. The officiate (in this case, the surgeon) will give you sacred instruction based on knowledge handed down through the generations, and you absorb the information on a level of trust. On the hero's journey, this dialogue is a classic interaction between the internal psyche and external archetypes. This type of interaction is described by Martin Buber, an Austrian-born Israeli philosopher.[43] He depicted relationships as "living" in the sacred space between people. The dialogue you share with your physician and your partner creates an energetic "living" agreement and understanding. Your intentions for the upcoming surgery are, in a sense, living in this space between the three of you.

Tests and Sacrifices

With the ritual of informed consent finalized, you will be ready for surgical preparation and may be asked to sacrifice some of your blood or urine for tests. You may also undergo a test called a radiograph or electrocardiogram to determine the health of your lungs and heart. A radiograph, or x-ray, checks to see if there is a lung mass or other anomaly that might make anesthesia difficult. An electrocardiogram determines the functionality of the heart's conduction system.

Blood is part of many rituals, including Christian Communion, in which participants voluntarily drink wine or juice as a vestige of Christ's blood. This ritual brings the congregation into a communion with themselves and with Christ and reminds them of life, death, and resurrection. This most sacred ritual involves symbolic blood of the Christian Savior because blood is a revered essence of life and death. When Jesus gives his disciples the cup and says, "Drink from it, all of you. This is the blood of my covenant, which is poured out for many for the forgiveness of sins"

(Matthew 26:26–28, New International Version), blood is being utilized to signify life and for a cleansing of the spirit. A blood test is asked of all preoperative patients to make sure they are physically prepared for the surgical process.

Another aspect of preparing for the ritual of surgery is continuity between the pre-surgery preparations, the surgery itself, and post-operative procedures. The importance of continuity in ritual is seen in the Kiowa Gourd Dance, which depicts the cycle of departure and return. In this story-dance about continuity, a young man was separated from his tribe and running out of food and water. Suddenly, he heard music coming from over a hill and saw a red wolf singing and dancing while on its hind legs. The wolf asked the young man to take the dance back to his tribe, and the howling at the end is tribute to the wolf that brought this man back to his community. And this ritualistic dance connects Kiowa Indians to their community.[44]

In addition to the blood sacrifice, surgery also requires a time sacrifice. If you know you will be having a C-section in advance, you and your surgeon can agree on a date that works well for both of you. If your surgical window is a couple weeks wide, you may be able to choose a day or date that appeals to you or avoid a date that doesn't. Carol was thrilled to schedule her C-section on St. Patrick's Day and named her son after the saint. Veronica wanted to avoid having her C-section on Friday the thirteenth. And Kelly said, "Any day this child is born will be a blessed day!" The sacredness of the time and dates selected is essential for the social support of the patient and expands their spiritual understanding of healing from a ancestral perspective.[45]

Fasting

During the twelve hours before surgery, you will be abstaining from food and drinking only water. If you've never fasted before, this may sound unpleasant, but if you stay centered and grounded, it can be a transcendent experience. Focus on nourishing yourself with music, beautiful images, and books or articles that inspire you. The transitional space between the preoperative phase and the C-section is bridged by the quiet of fasting.

Fasting also bridges religious worlds. Along with prayer, chanting, study of sacred texts, worship, and ordinances,[46] fasting is a common spiritual practice for individuals setting a sacred space. The fasting you do before your C-section will help to reduce your stomach acid and thus the likelihood of aspiration during surgery.[47] But rest assured that most women don't experience any nausea during this surgical process and are completely awake. For those unfortunate few who might experience mild nausea, there are safe medications that will relieve this sensation almost immediately.

· · · · · · · · · · · · · · · · · · · ·

Journaling Cue: Write in your journey book frequently during the waking hours of your fast. What are you feeling? What emotions or memories are coming up? With the inner chatter of what to eat and when to eat silenced, what are the dominant thoughts filling your mind?

If the idea of fasting gives you pause, gain strength from the knowledge that fasting and other dietary rules are incorporated into many sacred rituals. For instance, in Vietnamese culture, women wishing to regain strength and vitality after childbirth while breastfeeding are asked to partake in a sacred ritual where they must adhere to a strict postnatal diet that prohibits fish, seafood, duck, and all meat except lean pork.[48]

The final process of the preoperative ritual and transition to the sacred space of the operating room is removing all vestiges of the outside world. You will remove your clothes, makeup, jewelry, nail polish, and any other external decorations and place them in a bag in the preoperative unit. This nakedness is a symbolic representation of the circle of life—both grave and womb.[49]

Preparing the Surgical Altar

Prior to being escorted to surgery, the surgical suite is prepared. The air filters are sterilizing and purifying the air. Sterile water and saline are poured into heated basins, and the process of counting begins. Trays of instruments are opened, and each has its sacred place on the operating room table.

Each surgeon has a card dictating what they want to have on this table for a C-section, and the scrub nurse prepares the table according to her specified ritual. It's important to see this process as the beginning of a circle. As each instrument, sponge, and needle is counted and subsequently used, the process will end according to these same sacred numbers. If the numbers at the beginning and ending of the surgery do not match precisely, then the surgery cannot end.

Another important part of the surgical ritual is purified water. Sacred ceremonies frequently include purified water, and the shaman or officiate will often carry a sacred bag filled with instruments of their trade.[50] These bags carry special objects of power like eagle feathers or personal items infused with power, and they can be called many names, such as the "muvieri" in Huichol customs. The muvieri itself is touched to all things owned by the healer and consecrated with blood, as are all the tools placed inside.[51] The shaman will also carefully lay their items out on a special blanket and place them in a formation specific to their needs; they may be scraps of cloth or instruments, but each is infused with power and necessary for the healing process.[52] The point of preparation for a sacred process is that each item has its place. The item may not be used, but it will go back to the bundle or back to central supply, where it will be sterilized until needed again.

The final piece of surgical suite preparation is counting the instruments and sponges. This process is so sacred that it takes place three times during the surgery, with the following criteria: those individuals counting must remain the same, the counts must match each time, the fatigue of the participants is noted, and the urgency of the procedure changes the manner in which items are counted.[53] Items are counted before, during, and at the end of the procedure; this counting may be one of the most revered parts of the surgical process.

Once the surgical altar is properly prepared, you will be brought to the room in an altered state of consciousness, having been given a sedative or painkillers prior to the transition. Once again, your path mirrors the epic hero's journey, as the hero must be altered prior to entering this sacred space.

Entering the Extraordinary World

The world of most surgical suites is awash in light blue or green caps, gowns, and scrubs. Although some hospitals are moving away from the classic blue and green color scheme for the operating room, we like it. The color blue is "linked with eternity, the beyond, supernatural beauty, religious transcendence, the spiritual and mental as contrasted with the emotional and physical and with detachment from the earthly."[54] Before the ritual can begin, your belly will be cleansed with an antiseptic, and a narrow plastic tube called a catheter will be inserted into your bladder. Sterile drapes will frame your abdomen and may be hung on a bar between your chest and your hips to block your view. But don't worry! You will still get to see your baby the moment he or she is delivered. While you are draped in covers and the surgical instruments are waiting on a sterile surgical field, your surgeon is outside cleansing their hands. This scrubbing is obviously functional for antisepsis, but it also serves a ritualistic purpose.

As in baptism, physical cleansing has been a part of sacred ceremonies for millennia. In many sacred ceremonies there is a connection between the physical purity and the moral purity of the ritual—in a sense a washing away of sins prior to the procedure.[55] Once the hands and forearms are cleansed, the surgeon and their assistant enter the room with hands held away from the body. This process of entering the room with the patient prepared is synonymous with the surgeon preparing to enter the healing plane and the patient's physical body. Gowns are donned, and the surgeon prepares to make the incision.

As in many sacred rituals, your name and the name of the procedure will be called out by the circulating nurse before the surgery begins. This naming of patient and procedure is called a "time out" in the operatory and is required by medical governing bodies, but it can also serve as a preparatory pause.[56] In the allopathic realm, this "time out" is a means for the participants to unify the right patient and the right surgery. In a ritualistic sense, this "preparatory pause" adds a level of mindfulness to focus on you and the procedure at hand. The theater is ready, the participants are in place, and it is now time for the heart of the ritual to begin.

From the Sacred Wound, New Life Springs Forth

Most women are happy to know that the surgical incision is usually a horizontal line, sometimes called a "bikini cut," made right above your pubic hairline. So while the wound is sacred, the scar will not be very noticeable after it heals. In the case of a C-section, the sacred wound is an incision made to lift your baby from the internal world of your womb to the outside world. In order to do this, another incision is made in your uterus. Your baby will then be carefully lifted up and out. Their mouth and nose will be suctioned out, and you'll hear baby's first cry. You will get to see the baby for a moment and may even get to hold them for a few minutes, but that will depend on your medical condition and hospital protocol. If you have to wait to hold your baby, focusing on the spiritual bond that you've established over the past nine months will be a comfort for both of you.

Mythically, the wound as an opening is also a gateway to potential transformation and a window into encapsulated history.[57] In many instances, the wound is created by a wounded healer or a surgeon who carries their own scars. In Shawn's mythology, through genograms he discovered that all maternal relationships in his family were connected by conflict. When he saw this conflict on paper, he understood that the reason he became a gynecologist, specifically choosing to care for mothers and women, was complex and deeply informed by this conflict. It was through maturation and discovery that he was able to become a better physician and wrestle with these inner demons.

In ritualistic indigenous cultures, the first stage to becoming a healer is that of the calling[58]; this call can come from the family, the community, or from the world beyond. Shamans are called and then receive rigorous instruction, followed by initiation and practice. Allopathic physicians have similar stages of development: the call to be a physician, followed by the structured education of medical school, the initiation of residency, and ultimately the practice of medicine in the community.[59] Healers may have emotional, physical, or mental challenges that result in a spiritual insight or awareness that comes once they've surrendered to their own wounds; these wounds become part of the "medicine bundle," or tools, of the surgeon. Wounds are an essential piece of the healing ceremony because without wounds there would be no reason to heal. The ritual of an operation commences before—sometimes long before—the incision is made, and it may continue for a long period after the wound is healed.[60]

In between the beginning and end points of the ritual is the spiritual process of entering another's physical body. This spiritual process of knowing the patient as a person builds a powerful bond between care provider and patient, increasing patient advocacy when they are under anesthesia.[61] Experiencing the patient externally and internally is the basis for this person-centered ritual of surgery, and continuity of care is essential for ongoing psychological support from a spiritual perspective.[62]

All women begin their pregnancies with the hope that surgical intervention won't be needed. As doctors and parents, that is also our hope, and together with our expectant moms we set the intention for a safe, smooth delivery. But when circumstances dictate assisting the birth with an intervention or with a cesarean section, we are always relieved and grateful that we have this option to save the baby's life without compromising the mother's. And whether you deliver your baby or your doctor performs a C-section, your baby's transition from your sacred womb to your loving arms will stop time and change your life forever.

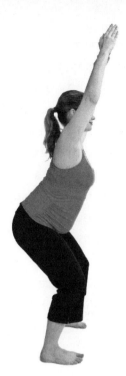

Yoga Pose
Chair Pose
Settling In

This standing pose will strengthen your core muscles and your leg muscles and improve your balance. You may find it easier to do in shallow water, particularly during the third trimester. The water's buoyancy will naturally displace your weight, cradling you as you move. Moving in water also aids oxygen efficiency.

Stand with your feet hip-distance apart. Gently straighten your lower back by slightly bending your knees and tipping your pelvic bones up in the front. If your pelvis were a bowl filled with water, this position would keep the water from spilling out in front of you.

Bend your knees farther, as if you're about to sit in a chair.

Roll your shoulders back and down.

Lift up your arms and reach for the stars.

While in this position, take several full breaths. As you inhale, let your belly expand. As you inhale, pull your belly in.

Benefits

- Chair Pose reminds us to settle into our bodies, relax in the face of discomfort, and let go of the things we can't control.

Precautions

- If you feel out of balance going into this pose, stop and use a strong handhold.

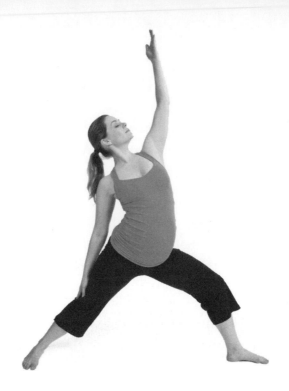

Yoga Pose
Reverse Warrior
Exaltation and Gratitude

Begin in Warrior II position (see page 110) and bring your front arm straight up, lengthening your torso and keeping a bend in your front knee.

Place your back hand on your back thigh. Breathe and hold for two to three breaths. Focus on your breath and notice your arm lifting as your front knee bends.

Benefits
- This pose can inspire you and fill you with gratitude, keeping you grounded in the moment.

Precautions
- If you feel unsteady, modify this pose by holding onto a chair or the wall with your back hand instead of placing it on your back thigh.

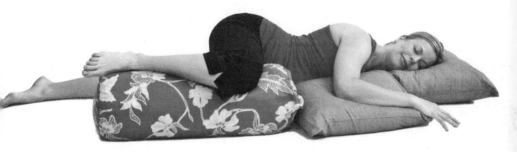

Yoga Pose
Corpse Pose
Relaxation and Relief

Corpse Pose is one of the most relaxing poses in yoga and can be done at any stage in the pregnancy, after childbirth, and after a C-section. It is a wonderful pose for increasing your inner awareness and staying in touch with yourself as the baby takes center stage.

Lie on your right or left side with a bolster or blanket between your knees, and focus your attention on your breath.

Slowly bring your attention to your thoughts. As those thoughts enter your mind like a butterfly landing in your hands, allow them to take off and gently drift away; let them come and go.

Where does your body feel most relaxed right now? Wherever it is most relaxed, imagine that relaxation spreading throughout your entire body.

Familiarize yourself with this sense of deep relaxation, and each time you enter this pose go deeper into the surrender and deeper into this ability of letting go.

On your hero's journey, giving birth is the most physically and emotionally challenging stage. This is where you stand in your strength and use everything that you've learned to help your baby begin their own journey in this world. If this were a movie, the audience would be holding their collective breath until they hear your baby take his or her first breath and cry. In real life, you will likely have that same reaction, but the anxious feeling will quickly be overtaken by extreme joy. When your eyes behold your beloved baby, the Holy Grail, for the first time, your heart will soar with joyful bliss that only a mother knows. You will have triumphed in your goal to bring this new spirit safely into the world. Your heart will sing as your partner and all of your loved ones celebrate this miraculous new life.

In your journey to motherhood, you've conquered the darkness of your fears: pain and doubt. And now it is time to return to your "ordinary" world, bringing with you a higher knowledge or purpose and your precious baby. You reenter this world as a changed woman. The previous nine months have been about you and the life growing inside you—an internal focus and preparation for the next leg of this amazing journey. And your new journey has already begun; it began the moment you gave birth and gazed for the first time into your baby's eyes.

Part 5
Beyond Birth

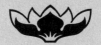

The Road Back

In lore and literature, the last cycle of a journey or pilgrimage is sometimes described as the road back because the hero begins to move back toward real life or what's sometimes called the ordinary world. But she has been changed by the journey and is no longer the woman she was when she set out. She's stronger, braver, and wiser, and she brings with her a magical gift, prize, or achievement. For you, this magical gift is your baby.

Brava! You have successfully completed your hero's journey through your spiritually aware pregnancy and childbirth. Without a doubt, you now understand how nine months of gestation initiates mothers into a deep understanding of the journey's process. Growth is process. Birth is process. Even cooking, that most humble and exalted of art forms, is a process. During your pregnancy, and again during the birthing process, you learned that nature has her own time schedule and plan. No amount of wishing on your part could rush the process. Instead, you had to adjust to dealing with "what is" at any given moment and be able to release control to the powers that be. Your journey opened your heart to a greater understanding of the dynamic of creation in all its incarnations and everyday manifestations.

Chapter 9

Life after Birth

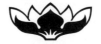

I love them (my boys) and their
births that brought them to me, but
I also love how giving birth to them
allowed me to grow as a woman.
Ricki Lake, *Your Best Birth*

When mothers describe the days following the births of their children, they use words like surreal, magical, and overwhelming. Lynn, a twenty-eight-year-old new mother, said that when she returned home with baby Christine,

> Everything was different, at least slightly. Surreal, new, overwhelming in some ways, but good. Amazing, too, how quickly it became the norm, in that it felt like she'd always been a part of our lives. Thinking back, trying to remember, even now, she's somehow part of the memories of "life before baby." Once my parents left, I couldn't believe how little free time there was in the day. But it was wonderful, relaxing in a way, to be home with my baby. It was also great to be able to hunker down to recover physically and

bond emotionally with my husband, Dave, and with Christine. Getting back to anything resembling a normal routine took a while! I am so grateful for my mom's help and for everyone who brought us meals...not having to cook was a lifesaver!

Our friend Margaret said she was so mesmerized by her daughter Bella in the days after her birth that it was hard for her to do anything but focus on her. She said:

> I was so taken by her presence those first few days that I couldn't focus on anything else. Funny thing, I didn't brush my teeth for a couple of days, and didn't even notice until my mom came to visit. It wasn't so much that my ordinary world looked different, it was that I felt so different...so connected to this person I knew in my belly during pregnancy who was now looking at me and had needs and wants I had never addressed with anyone before. I didn't want to focus on anything but our relationship. I remember we didn't venture out of the house for two weeks, and after that, we sat on the porch for the first few days, and then finally took a walk around our neighborhood with her in the stroller. During those two weeks in the house, I felt like we were in a bubble, a love bubble...very sweet. On a practical note, my labor was long, and I appreciated any rest I got those first few days (which wasn't much).

The after-birth transformation that new mothers experience is noticeable and lasting. This powerful shift in the outer world follows in the wake of your shedding the placenta, or afterbirth, from baby's inner world.

The Power of the Placenta

The miraculous afterbirth, so called because it comes out of the womb after birth, is a blood- and nutrient-rich organ connected to the uterine wall. The word *placenta* comes from the Latin meaning "flat cake." As we've mentioned, the placenta delivered nutrients and oxygen from your body to your baby while you were pregnant. It also churned out powerful hormones, including progesterone, estrogen, and relaxin. In a real sense, the placenta is an inner guardian angel, secreting oxytocin—which eases birth stress—and a molecule called placental opioid-enhancing factor (POEF) that encourages a natural reduction in pain during and after delivery.

Even after its natural expulsion from your body, the placenta is viewed by many cultures as spiritually powerful. From the dawn of time, world cultures have viewed the placenta as a tie that binds mother and child to the spirit realm. Many world cultures still view the afterbirth as a vehicle for the soul essence of a baby. It is sometimes even regarded as the baby's twin or guardian spirit. Modern mothers are coming to see the placenta in the same spiritual light as many of these global cultures. For the past fifty years, hospitals routinely have been disposing of the placenta as "medical waste" or have been selling it to companies that use its dense nutrients as base matter for a variety of products. Today, the sale of placentas by hospitals is declining, and part of the reason is the increasing understanding of its cultural and spiritual significance. Right now, there are no universal standards for placenta disposal, but new mothers should ask their hospitals about procedures, as standards vary across the country.

In many cultures worldwide (particularly the Aboriginal cultures of Australia and certain groups in Africa), the placenta is revered, sometimes as a twin of the child and sometimes as an arbiter of the child's fate. Consequently, the placenta is usually buried or disposed of in a highly ritualistic way. In ancient Egypt, the pharaoh's placenta was considered his twin and was preserved and brought into battle on a long stick.

Some modern-day African cultures still have the same time-honored belief and follow elaborate spiritual practices designed to ensure the spirit "twin" helps the child from the spirit realm in auspicious ways.

Placenta Trees

In Central Africa, the Baganda people put the afterbirth in a pot and bury it under a plantain tree. The tree is watched carefully lest anyone eat from it and scare the twin spirit away. It is also thought that if animals eat from the tree, the human child may take on spiritual or physical values of those animals.

Australian Aboriginal cultures also practice afterbirth rituals with special family trees. Some groups have buried placentas under certain trees designated for their families for centuries. The trees then become a living part of the blood, tissue, spirit, and generational history of that family. The rise of a global web-based culture has led spiritually curious new parents (including some high-profile celebrities) to adopt this ancient practice and bury placentas under their own special placenta tree. Less popular is the practice of eating the placenta, a ritual that has some basis in nutritional theory (some say the nutrients in the placenta help the mother with postpartum depression). This may sound disgusting, but it's the most natural thing in the world for nearly all the other mammals, so it seems they know something that we don't know. Eating the placenta may replace important nutrients lost during pregnancy and childbirth, and it may also prevent postpartum depression. Though this has yet to be scientifically proven, there are many well-respected midwives that promote the use of encapsulated placenta to cure everything from depression to anemia.

If you're planning your own placenta tree ritual, we urge you to speak to your admitting hospital or ob-gyn first. If the hospital where you're delivering allows patients to take home a placenta, you must follow their instructions about storage (freezing is usually necessary to prevent germs growing and spreading). The placenta is not considered human remains and so it is legal to bury it, but in some cases your care provider may need to biopsy the organ after birth. If HIV or other infectious agents are present, it is against public safety regulations to take it home.

Lotus Birth

Some cultures (Aboriginal tribes in Australia and the Balinese) and some sects of Christians and Jews believe in allowing the afterbirth and umbilical cord to fall away on its own, a practice called "Lotus Birth" or umbilical nonseverance. Lotus Birth is practiced by some birthing centers as well as by some home-birthing facilitators. As you probably surmised, this is not a common practice in American hospitals.

The process relies on presumed changes that produce internal clamping within ten to twenty minutes after a woman gives birth. Over the next ten to fourteen days, the umbilical cord dries to a sinew and naturally detaches from the baby's belly button. Detachment generally occurs two to three days after birth. Believers in the procedure say it can prevent breastfeeding jaundice and loss of healthy birth weight, although we don't have scientific evidence to support this yet. Because of standardized medical protocol, most hospitals don't offer this option.

Healing Body, Mind, and Spirit

Many non-Western world cultures have very specific 30–40 day resting rituals designed to help new mothers restore body and spirit after birth. Around the world, forty days is also the standard length of time for a life-changing spiritual practice. In Hindu practice, one prays using mala beads for a period of forty days. In Christian practice, there are the forty days of Lent and Jesus's forty days in the wilderness. These rituals designate the time after birth as a special and vulnerable space for the new mother. In Guatemala, a new mother rests for twenty days, supported by friends and family, kept warm and well fed; at the end of that time, she is given a ritual soboda, a postpartum massage/bath by the midwife, which is said to help her produce milk and which formally and ritualistically ends the birth process.

The Chinese custom of *zuo yue zi* ("doing the month") dictates that new mothers should not walk outside, read, cry, bathe, wash her hair, touch cold water, or engage in sexual intercourse in the month after birth. The belief is that it is very important for new mothers to keep warm and to be protected from the wind element, which could harm the body by entering joints.

In India and North Africa, the forty-day rest period includes the ornate and beautiful ritual of henna—the red dyes derived from the henna plant—now familiar to Western women as body ornamentation and offered in many mainstream spas and salons. In its traditional form, the intricate designs plied on the skin with the natural henna dye are meant to protect the new mother and to seal in the magic, or *baraka*, that the process of birthing creates. In Rajisthan, this ritual is called "the filling of the lap." The new mother is seated on a special throne, and family and friends fill her lap with sweets, fruits, and a coconut.

The use of henna after giving birth is a particularly feminine ritual done by women for women. Women sit with the new mother and design the intricate patterns of dye on the body, which can take hours to paint and to dry. During this time, the mother cannot use her hands lest she ruin the patterns on her hands and fingers. Friends and family feed her, brush her hair, and make her comfortable. After the dye is set, the forty-day fast from chores and regular life ensure the patterns (and good luck) stay visible. This time also ensures that the mother feels a special separate healing space during which she can restore her body (nutrient-rich meats are often fed to mothers during this time) and bond with her baby without the distractions of life interfering.

This ritual bears similarities with a ritual done by certain groups of Buddhists in Laos for a person who has just finished a long journey. The belief is that the soul becomes vulnerable during travel, and parts of it are leaked out and need to be brought back to make the person whole again. After prayers are said to call these soul parts back, wrists are bound with white lambswool to help the person retain their wandering spirit. Shamans have a similar tradition of soul retrieval after physically or mentally momentous events or traumas.

Pregnancy is one of the most meaningful journeys a woman can take. If you consider that your mind, body, and spirit need time to center (much as the traveler does in Laotian Buddhist thought), you can tap in to your own tradition and culture to give yourself the time and space you need to rest, restore, and collect yourself before you move back into the world of everyday life. One of the most centering things you can do is to work with the lessons you've learned through nine months of a spiritually aware pregnancy.

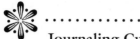

Journaling Cue: Take out your journey book and write about the changes you've undergone in these past magical months. They will continue to transform you in the days, months, and years to come.

Life Lessons from Your Epic Journey

Ricki Lake's film *The Business of Being Born* includes interviews with many recent mothers (as well as midwives) on the transformational experience of giving birth. Many of these women mention the same processes and spiritual transformations that we hear over and over from our patients. Women talk about owning the process of childbirth, the necessity of trust, the feeling of oneness with a universal concept of motherhood. And they talk about reaching a point in the birthing process where they thought they couldn't do it—and then they did! This is the classic experience of cresting the summit in your hero's journey.

The birth of a baby can feel like an impossible rock and a hard place at the end of a long journey. On the one side is the pain of pushing and the thought that "this is impossible," and on the other is the deep drive to move beyond the pain, around it, or inside it. On the other side of that seemingly impenetrable wall is a miracle: life! The ecstasy and love hormone oxytocin (the same one released in orgasm) floods the new mother's body, sugarcoating the pain of childbirth with joy. You can't separate the orgasmic ecstasy from the pain. They are yin and yang, one and the same thing, or, as we say in Western society, two sides of the same coin.

When you push beyond that wall, you learn that many barriers you believed were insurmountable can be leapt over in a single bound. Like many new mothers, you may be thinking, "If I can do this, I can do anything!" You have also gained a new understanding of pain that only women who have given birth can know. As the natural human feeling of pain as a barrier disappeared, it was replaced by an abiding strength and the wisdom that pain is a threshold to be crossed—a threshold that binds all mothers to all mothers before them.

Trust and Surrender

Ask any new mother about trust and surrender, and a wealth of experiences, thoughts, and memories will flood forth. At the beginning of a hero's journey there is always doubt, insecurity, and unspoken fears. The spiritually aware mother-to-be may have many moments of letting go and learning to trust the process. There may be the need to recommit to trust over and over again. There may even be a point where old ideas, fears, and beliefs are challenged.

Laundry lists are drawn up and some of these old items may be discarded in the surrender process. You really wanted a boy and you found out you were having a girl. Or you wanted a girl and you've got twin boys! Some new mothers find that the type of birthing experience they counted on was not the optimal choice for the health of the mother and baby. Other mothers experience high-risk pregnancies that require bed rest or other major changes. But all mothers learn to surrender to the process that makes the best sense for both mother and child.

Zen Buddhists believe in the growth power of right action. Doing good works or "right actions" is said to be the same as planting seeds of enlightenment, and along your hero's journey you have planted many seeds. Spiritual pregnancies are seeds of faith in action. And through the nine months and giving birth, you have harvested a cornucopia of spiritual truths that will serve you forever.

Perfect Love

A spiritually aware pregnancy naturally leads you to understand perfection in new ways. We've assisted hundreds of births where the phrase "She's perfect!" is exclaimed at the moment when the baby is placed on the mother's breast. This perfection is not based on the fact that the mother has just given birth to a poster child, destined to become the next Gerber baby. This perfection is based on the perfect moment of love and bonding that never fails to move us.

Spiritually aware moms can internalize that understanding of "perfect" and turn it inward—especially just after pregnancy—to themselves. Seeing their post-pregnancy bodies with the same love, they can say, "I'm perfect! It's me and it's perfect for right now." Buddhism views the conception of perfection in this way. Many Buddhist teachings exhort believers to understand the universe and themselves as being perfect as they are. This does not mean that you cannot exert change or make things better in the world. It means viewing what is for exactly what it is, not what you wish it to be.

Surmounting the Rock and a Hard Place

In the early days of the resurgence of natural childbirth in the 1960s, women talked about the pain as fading once you held the baby in your arms. Women would advise each other, "It hurts like hell, but all that pain fades when the baby comes out." In earlier generations when women were put into the "twilight sleep" of scopolamine, they literally did not remember the pain they experienced during labor. This is no longer viewed as a good thing. In the hero's journey, the Holy Grail, the ultimate boon, is achieved only after the darkness of pain, doubt, fear, and fatigue are conquered. Forgetting that journey is not being a spiritually aware hero; internalizing the journey and the victory over darkness is.

Hindu culture has a wonderful image of a mother who has conquered fear and darkness: Durga (sometimes called Durga Ma). In Sanskrit, *Durga* means a fort or a place that is difficult to overrun. Durga is the slayer of the demon that represents all evils, especially our inner demons of anger, fear, hate, and lust. She embodies Shakti, the mother/female force of the world. She is the ultimate spiritual mother, and she is often pictured riding on a lion or tiger—illustrating the concept that she has conquered darkness through power, will, and determination. During the yearly ten-day Durga festival, Hindus practice a variety of rituals and speak and chant mantras designed to honor their strong mother icon. One of these mantras is "Jai Ma," which is Sanskrit for "victory to the Divine Mother."

We would like to suggest that you say "Jai!" ("Victory!") to the new mother you've just brought into the world along with your new baby. This positive exclamation does not negate or diminish the twists and turns of the road ahead. There are likely to be plenty of them. But you'll have your pilgrim's pack from your nine-month journey into yourself and into the very heart of motherhood. This pack contains resources of heightened awareness and spiritual skills you'll be able to count on in everyday life and through the lifelong journey of motherhood.

Journeywork
Creating Your
"New You" Vision Board

Whether you're a new mother for the first time or the fifth, the experience has deepened and transformed you. Now's the perfect time to create a physical representation of your vision for the road ahead. You may be familiar with the concept of the vision board or life map collage popularized by Oprah Winfrey and other life coaches. By creating a vision board of yourself as a new mother, you can begin to clarify who you are now and what you would love to manifest on the road ahead. The process is simple and fun.

Collect a good amount of magazines and newspapers with images that you can cut out.

Gather your supplies: a large poster board, scissors, and clear glue that will not soak through and stain the fronts of the images you choose.

Find a quiet place to sit. Play calming music or listen to the sounds of nature.

Flip through the magazines and newspapers and cut out anything that appeals to you for any reason. Don't think about it too much. Let your impulse be your guide.

Now, glue the images onto the board wherever and however it feels right to you. (There is no wrong way to do this.) You can also write on your board and use glitter, stickers, fabric swatches, or other touches that express your feelings about yourself as a new mother. Don't censor yourself.

When you're finished, put the board away for a few days. Then retrieve it and sit in front of it for about fifteen minutes. Don't judge the images you selected, just take them in. If there is something you want to add to the board, feel free to do so.

Your vision board can be put away and looked at from time to time or displayed in a place where you see it often and can use it to meditate on your highest good and your best self as a new mom.

Life with Baby

For forty weeks you imagined her every time you felt a kick or pictured him every time you felt the gentle ripple as he moved a foot, swimming in his pool of amniotic fluid. You were filled with anticipation and the impossible expectations of what you might feel and what you would experience from the moment you beheld her or held him in your arms.

And now the time to take your precious baby home has finally arrived. But with this juncture, many new mothers also have a flurry of worries and anxieties as the words "now what?" crowd their consciousness. Even as you learn how to hold baby, wrap him, change her diaper, and nurse, you are in a daze. You're blissed out by love for this new little being—and at the same time you may be overwhelmed by the terror of it all. The challenge of returning from a heroic quest is retaining what you've learned on the way. Now is the time to integrate your deeper understanding of yourself and the world—and bring this understanding into your everyday life as time moves forward.

Just as you were assisted by helpers and guides on your pregnancy journey, you can reach out for guidance and support on your new path of everyday life. Everyday life is altered now—in some ways temporarily and others irrevocably. Physically you are still healing, but your schedule seems to have little time for rest or recovery. Your baby needs you. How can you manage with all that is new, all that is changed? You have the tools—acquired during the past nine months—to draw upon, and you are ready.

The coming days, weeks, and months will be a journey of firsts: from his first smile to her first words to his first steps. Each day, even the ones when you're exhausted, will be filled with wonder and amazement. Just as every journey on your life's path will enlighten the next, the wisdom, knowledge, and deeper awareness of yourself and your environment that you've acquired during your pregnancy and childbirth can inform the days ahead as you return from your largely internal odyssey into the real world. You have emerged the hero of this nine-month journey, and while in some ways you are the same woman you've always been, in other ways you have been irrevocably altered.

Margaret shared, "As far as returning to a routine after giving birth, 'nothing has felt the same' may sound cliché, but I felt made new—in challenging and supportive ways."

Today Margaret is the mom of six-year-old Bella and three-year-old Kirsten. She says that once she had children, she never again felt the way she did before she had them:

> I felt grounded in who I was before I had my children, so I didn't think there would be such a dramatic transformation. My essence hasn't changed one bit, but my approach to life on earth has and my experience of space and time surely has. One thought that came to me shortly after Bella was born and has remained with me throughout is that my experience of having children, being a mom, has brought me into the now, the present moment, in a whole new way. Having children yanked me into the present moment so that I am in it more consistently than I used to be. No

more "checking out" for periods of time, no long breaks, or short ones, from what Life is putting in front of me. This is my greatest blessing and has brought out my greatest challenges.

Like Margaret and all new mothers, during your pregnancy you learned to understand the spiritual being within and place it in harmony with the new life that was growing inside you. Now it is time to take hold of the gifts acquired during this time and bring them into your new place of being. The ability to bring the spiritual into the new world, with its new challenges, will allow you to find amazement and a sense of the miraculous in even the most challenging moments of parenthood.

Like the hero of a classic tale, you must now cross a threshold back into an altered reality, changed by the journey you've just been through. Life is altered both by the presence of your baby and by the physical, emotional, and spiritual changes you've gone through on your quest.

 . . . .

Journaling Cue: How can I retain the self-aware, internal wisdom I acquired and integrate that into this next phase of living—this new quest or journey into parenthood? How do I embrace the challenges along with the joys—the mundane tasks along with the breathtaking amazement of new parenthood?

It is possible to bring the spiritual experience along with you as you reenter your daily life, which will now include the rituals of parenting a newborn. You can maintain a stubborn hold on your sacred spaces and create magnificent pools of sacred time— time set aside for you apart from your baby to breathe, to rest, to reenergize. Life is as much about separation—creating divisions between things—as it is about joining together. We need to live in both zones, and maintaining a sense of the sacred will help you endure the toughest moments and perhaps allow you to sense the Divine even in those.

You might have imagined during your pregnancy what it would be like to bring home your newborn. If it is your first child, your imagination may have run wild with idyllic visions unhindered by experience (no matter what you might have been warned by friends and family). It's not uncommon to underestimate the challenges you now face because you typically have to experience this stage of life before you can truly comprehend it. It's also not uncommon to underestimate the incredible, the awesome, and the amazing that you are about to experience every day, over and over again. Finding the harmony between the two—finding balance between the challenges and the joys—is key to walking the road ahead. There will be times when it feels more like walking a tightrope than a road and you'll want to flee, to return to the beauty of dreams and imaginings. But one look at your beautiful baby and thoughts of fleeing will be replaced with a depth of love that fills you from your head to your toes.

Seeing the World Through Baby's Eyes
Our friend Carol shared a wonderful story of how she learned to see the world through her baby's eyes. She said:

> I remember one day when Ellie was a few months old, I went into the nursery to pick her up after her nap and she was staring at the ceiling. When I called her name, she didn't look at me, and my heart stopped for a second. I thought something was terribly wrong. Finally I followed her eyes to the ceiling and saw a patch of dancing white

lights. The reflection of water dripping into a puddle outside the nursery was creating this display, and Ellie was mesmerized. I'd lived in the house for two years and I'd never noticed the dancing lights on the ceiling.

Babies have a magical way of helping us to see the world through their eyes. The spiritual journey of pregnancy and childbirth will allow you to tune in to what your baby is seeing and pay attention to whatever holds their interest. Everyday objects will take on new dimensions as you imagine what they must look like to baby. Everyday events that you have been taking for granted, like the sun streaming through your kitchen window, will be rediscovered and appreciated anew as you notice baby looking in wonderment at this beam of light. By watching your baby, you can don "baby-colored glasses" and find beauty in everything you see. With this perspective, your spirit will be touched by even the smallest things.

Babies are curious about everything they see, hear, taste, touch, and smell. Following their lead, learn to find the *wow* in what your baby senses. Let yourself experience their sense of wonder for yourself, putting you in tune with the world around you in a way that hasn't happened since you were a child yourself. This "second childhood" has the power to open the gateway to the divine love that you have for your baby and for your parents, even if your relationship with them was difficult. By following your baby's lead, you will be led through a process of rediscovery. By letting your baby be your guide, you can then be theirs as well.

It is a gift to be able to find moments of awe as only a child can when they experience something for the first time. And it's not just the obvious: the blue of the sky, the grandeur of the mountains. The twentieth-century poet E. E. Cummings wrote:

> I thank You God for this most amazing day: for the leaping greenly spirits of trees and a blue true dream of sky; and for everything which is natural which is infinite which is yes.

What is it that your baby sees that she finds so fascinating? Is it the colorful fish in your aquarium she's following with her eyes as they dart from one end to the other, or is it some subtler mystery that's attracted her attention? Perhaps it's the way the light glints off the coral or illuminates the ripples in the water. Maybe it's that scratch in the glass you haven't noticed in ages (if ever).

To see how your baby sees, be in touch with your inner eye—that part you tapped into while you were pregnant that gave you heightened senses and a sense of wonder at what was happening inside you—the eye that saw in a spark of the Divine something extraordinary in everything.

Let "what's that?" become a regular part of your vocabulary. What do you see that has you so engaged, my child? Eventually your "what's that?" may become your child's too, asking you "what's that?" as they begin to verbalize their curiosity. Except it may not come out exactly as "what's that." Perhaps it only sounds like gibberish—"whaaazzzaaaah?" But if you listen with your custom-tuned parent ears, you'll discern the question and share in the joy of discovery and amazement. When you are in touch with how your baby sees the world, a flower becomes more than a flower—it becomes a rich and wondrous world of color, texture, scent, and life—something exquisite and divine.

Can you take wonder even further, transcending the moment to explore what lies beyond this singular moment—when wonder becomes awe? In his book *Who Is Man?*, Abraham Heschel defines awe as "the awareness of transcendent meaning, of a spiritual suggestiveness of reality (a sense that something lies behind and created the moment of wonder)…an answer of the heart and mind to the presence of mystery in all things, an intuition for a meaning that is beyond the mystery, an awareness of the transcendent worth of the universe." Let your new baby be your guide.

A Whole New World of Sound

Your baby not only uses their eyes to perceive the amazing world, each sense is put to use to discover and explore. Meanwhile, you are using your senses to understand your child's needs, delights, and discomforts. Sounds, sensations, scents (not always so pleasant), and tastes take on greater meaning and connect you to your newborn's world.

Every living thing has its own way of communicating. As a new parent you will soon be hearing with that special radar that is custom-tuned to your baby's unique frequency. You will know the crashing, resounding cymbals of his cries: tired, hungry, distressed, lonely—or in pain. Although your baby's cries will sometimes rattle your nerves, there are other sounds that will be music to your ears. You will know the harp sounds of her contentment, her coos, his distinct laughter, the percussion of her sighs, his snores. Since your new child can't yet talk, you have to learn his language quickly; it is articulate and forceful—and possibly as strange to your ears as any foreign tongue. But you will learn to speak her language soon enough!

But what does your newborn hear? Watch him as he responds to the sound of your voice. Listen to how she calms to the soothing lilt of your tone or giggles to the new sounds she experiences. Babies startle at unexpected noises, yelling, and chaos, but they love the sound of gentle music and the color and bounce of lively tunes. Sing to your child; babies are the most uncritical music critics in the world. To baby's ears, your voice is divine and sublime.

Have fun introducing baby to new sounds: a bird, the meow of your cat, the drone of a plane overhead as she becomes more accustomed to this new experience of hearing. Stop and listen for the melodies of your environment, perhaps as you never have before.

The Sublime Newness of Touch

Babies love to touch. They find fascination with the angles and planes of faces, eyeglasses, lips, noses—pretty much everything. Their tiny fingers reach out to explore and discover their new environment. They curl around your finger, they bat at your eyes, feel your hair, reach inside your mouth. What is he experiencing or seeking? Is the texture of your tongue fun to touch? Or is it the warmth of your mouth that she finds appealing? What is he trying to understand about this other being, known as "Mommy" or "Daddy"?

Touch is something we adults usually take for granted, but tactile sensations can connect us to the spiritual and lead us to awe as profoundly as the things we see. The softness of a puppy as we stroke her fur and feel the downiness and the warmth of her body throughout our fingertips brings pleasure and provides comfort. The velvet of a rose's petals feels sublime on the fingers; how awesome is the texture?

Then there is the feel of a baby—your new baby—cuddled close to you, warm and snug. It brings you pleasure, and the feeling is mutual. Touch, cradling, and cuddling is an absolute necessity for both you and your baby. We all need to be touched, held, cradled—even as adults. Babies love and need to be touched; it's how they connect with the new humans in their lives—how they bond with you. Babies cannot be held and cuddled too much. In many cultures and for many centuries, swaddling has been a crucial part of making a newborn feel safe, secure, loved, and touched.

Native American papooses, African slings, and complex or simple modern contraptions you can buy or create will keep your new baby bundled tightly and held close.

Journeywork
Swaddling as Loving Touch

Lay a square baby blanket on a flat surface in a diamond shape.

Fold down the top corner about six inches.

Place your baby on his back with his neck and shoulders on the fold.

Pull the corner near your baby's right hand across his body, and tuck the leading edge under his back on the left side under the arm.

Pull the bottom corner up over the baby's left shoulder, tucking the blanket (and his left arm) tightly in the left back.

Bring the left side of the fold down right under the baby's chin and then pull the last corner all the way around the baby, tucking it in his left side.

With your baby swaddled, cuddled close to you, you connect body to body and soul to soul—you are one with each other. As you swaddle your baby (or perhaps as you hold him afterward), you may wish to recite a special prayer or poem of your own, or the following psalm (adapted from Psalm 104):

Creator of all things, Divine Spirit, your touch illuminates the world, gives it texture and form, clothed in splendor, wrapped in the light of the world as in a garment, unfolding the heavens like a curtain.

Of course the most intimate time for touching each other comes with feeding time. If you are nursing, you and your baby are connected physically with each other as she draws milk from your breast. It is miraculous that a baby's nourishment is provided: a perfect food, breast milk is manna in liquid form.

It is a direct connection between the spiritual, you, and your child. Yes, it is biology, chemistry, and physics that creates the breast milk for your baby, broken down into polysaccharides and the physics of suckling, but it is more than that, and your sense of wonder may ask for more than science to explain the feeling in feeding. If you're bottle-feeding, the connection is just as profound as you hold your child close to you, cuddled in the crook of your arm against your chest. You watch his face as he hungrily sucks and listen to the satisfied sigh when finished.

Bath time also offers an abundance of sensory riches. Warm water, soft washcloths, the act of washing the creases and folds of your baby's skin—all can become sources of amazement. Observe her toes: tiny and fragile, delicate nails—and so soft. Observe his legs that kicked and prodded for all those months, distending your abdomen as they poked from within. Now they are round and chubby, soft, with nearly translucent skin as you gently wash them.

Move up your baby's body and observe this little person that you created in partnership with the Divine, a legacy that goes back to the beginning of time itself. See her abdomen, the belly button—a prominent souvenir of her everlasting connection to you. Touch the softness of her downy skin, the fragile capillaries, blue just beneath the surface. Feel her heart beating, her arms splashing. Is she remembering her pre-birth home in the amniotic fluid of your belly?

Letting Go of Chaos

While your new baby fills your life with discovery and awe, they can also turn your life topsy-turvy, taking your previously calm world and rendering it chaotic. Household chores get put on hold, dishes fill the sink, dust accumulates, and taking even a moment for yourself seems but distant memory. Your once-wide world has contracted to a small bubble containing you and your baby. Everything comes down to your baby's needs, and your baby needs your constant attention. Even when she's asleep, you may have a hard time resting yourself because you want to make sure you're ready to respond to her when she's up. What if she needs a change? What if he needs to eat (again)? What if she's ill?

Then there are the trickier problems. Your new baby's days and nights are reversed. She wants to stay up and dance the night away when you are drained and exhausted. During the day, when you're yearning for connection, all he wants to do is sleep. Or maybe she refuses to go to sleep unless she's being held and rocked or driven around the block fifty times. And some babies, particularly if they're colicky, never seem to want to sleep and spend most of their time crying in discomfort and pain. Typically these difficult challenges don't last very long, but don't hesitate to reach out to other mothers and your doctor or midwife for suggestions and support. There are many answers about your baby's care that will be intuitive or seem like common sense, but it's a myth that mothers suddenly have all the answers.

And please don't feel guilty about scheduling some "off time" for yourself. It will be good for you and great for baby. This is important because even when everything's going smoothly, you will probably feel somewhat overwhelmed by motherhood's routine demands. You may long for a walk, a cup of coffee with friends, or to be back at work with the adults in your life. These are all normal feelings, so be gentle with yourself.

On the other hand, if you have a sense of melancholy or sadness that you can't seem to shake, you may have the baby blues, characterized by the following:

- weepiness

- sadness

- mood swings

- irritability

- anxiety

- loneliness

- restlessness

- impatience

Most women feel symptoms of the baby blues—perhaps 70 to 80 percent of all new moms get them. Fortunately, this often passes in a week or so as your body adjusts to all the changes. If your symptoms are more severe and don't dissipate, you may be experiencing the more intense (and much less common) postpartum depression that 10 to 15 percent of women suffer. These symptoms may include:

- loss of appetite

- insomnia

- intense irritability and anger

- overwhelming fatigue

- loss of interest in sex

- lack of joy in life

- feelings of shame, guilt, or inadequacy

- severe mood swings
- difficulty bonding with the baby
- withdrawal from family and friends
- thoughts of harming yourself or the baby

Despite the high-profile media around postpartum depression (PPD) and the public debate between Brooke Shields and Tom Cruise about the use of antidepressants during PPD, most new moms have experiences that are completely free of this unique form of temporary darkness. And maybe that's why the mothers who do experience it often find it shameful. They feel they should be up and around and that they should be feeling more love and a deeper desire to bond with their new baby. Not feeling these warm emotions often increases a new mother's emotional conflict and shame, and that, in turn, can slow or stall the healing process. It's time to unmask this mystery. During PPD, the feelings of sadness and melancholy tend to drown out these warm and positive feelings. And since PPD is a natural healing process for many women, we encourage our patients to give themselves permission to feel the emotions. Their bodies are physiologically creating the chemicals to produce these emotions for a reason, and we believe the reason is to help the woman heal on physical and spiritual levels.

Your baby's well-being depends on your own health, whether physical or emotional. You need to find respite—time to relax, center, and reenergize. Clear your mind; reconnect with yourself. Although it can be easier said than done, do take some time off from the new baby routine. You must also sleep and eat often and let people care for and pamper you. Slow down! Yes, you are the hero returned from her journey, but you are not Superwoman. You cannot do it all at every moment of the day and night. Consider that it's as much for your new child as it is for yourself.

Come into the power you hold within your spirit—the female power that is uniquely yours. Find a quiet corner for yourself; you need time to center, close your eyes, and relax your shoulders.

Journeywork
Centering

Take several cleansing breaths—deep, slow, and relaxing—as you feel energy begin to flow through you. Imagine a focal point like a beach with the waves rolling gently onto the sand or perhaps a green meadow sprinkled with colorful flowers. Hold this visual image while you imagine a pleasing sound like a wind chime, the gentle fall of rain, or birdsong.

Let the energy of the image and the soothing sound nourish you and ease the discomfort you feel in your lower body: your abdomen, your groin, your thighs. Allow the fatigue of your swollen breasts to dissipate as you breathe, energizing your mind, body, and spirit. Do this for 5–10 minutes one or more times a day to spiritually energize and calm yourself.

You can also do this exercise by putting on headphones and listening to music as you hold your visual image in your mind. Music has the power to enfold, relax, and draw you away from other thoughts and into yourself. Pop in a CD that you love or create a soothing playlist on your iPod for this journeywork—anything that allows you to lose yourself for a while while your baby sleeps is perfect.

When you open your eyes, you may wish to read the following prayer (or another one that resonates deeply with you):

Grant me the ability to listen to the voice inside me. It dwells deep within: the divine spirit guides my hand when I'm tired, provides the spark when I feel uninspired, and helps me find my footing when I'm apt to stumble in the newness of the task.

Grant me the courage to trust the instincts that mothers have somehow found since the dawn of creation within their own existence. I call upon the wisdom of the ages, to my mother and hers before that, and all the way back to the original Divine Feminine.

Grant me the wisdom to find time for me: to rest when I am weary, to sleep when I am tired, to light the embers of my spirit when they wane, knowing it is not a luxury but a necessity to gird me for the hours, days, and weeks ahead.

Divine Spirit, do not let me stand beaten and battered by the countless manifestations of my own inadequacies as I embark on motherhood. Aid me in this quest. Help me to find satisfaction and a deep, abiding pleasure in all that I have, in all that I do, and in all that I am.

Motherhood is a time of wonder, curiosity, discovery, and amazement. And it's also a time of uncertainty and anxiety. Up to this moment you may have only imagined what it would be like—the victorious hero who has returned home to conquer the next quest. Relax into this new journey; draw on what you have learned to this point. Take deep breaths, continue your yoga practice, and focus on keeping your heart open to your child, your mate, and yourself. You are poised to experience "being present" at a new level, and you are blessed to experience more love than you thought your heart could hold.

Chapter 10

After Birth Recall

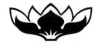

*In a child's eyes, a mother is a
goddess...I am convinced that this is
the greatest power in the universe.*
N. K. Jemisin,
The Hundred Thousand Kingdoms

One summer afternoon Shawn was driving our eight-year-old, Angelo, to basketball practice. He was at that stage of development where he'd talk from the backseat of the car and we'd learn all sorts of surprising information about him and his siblings. During this particular trip, from out of nowhere Angelo said, "Hey Dad, I remember being in Mom's belly."

Shawn was a little taken back, but was curious to hear what he had to say, so he said, "Really? What do you remember?"

He said, "Well, you know how if the sun is behind something like a piece of paper and you hold it up, you can see shadows? Well, I remember looking at the light coming through Mom's belly, and I could see her veins in a really neat pattern." He said all of this matter-of-factly.

"Wow—that sounds pretty cool."

Angelo was quiet for a couple minutes and then he dropped something on Shawn that surprised him even more.

He said, "It *is* cool, but that's not all. Sometimes the veins in Mom's belly turned into a picture of a face and talked to me while I was in there. They turned into the face of Buddha and told me to find my destiny."

Now it was Shawn's turn to be quiet—stunned, actually. Neither he or Katie are Buddhists. Katie did read books by notable authors such as Jon Kabat-Zinn and Jack Kornfeld and sometimes thought of Buddha when she was meditating or doing yoga during her pregnancy. Still, what eight-year-old talks about Buddha and finding his destiny?

There are two things that stand out from Angelo's bold statement. One is that he remembered seeing light in the uterus, and as we covered in part 3, researchers have shown that babies can detect light during the seventh month of pregnancy. The second is that he seems to have a recollection of messages or memories, and while this might be the topic for another book, we cannot discount this as simple imagination. Since that time he has purchased more than forty Buddha statues, which he has on display in our home. He also has Tibetan prayer flags hanging above the doorway to the room where he plays video games.

While Shawn was stunned when this occurred, he didn't discount the possibility of it being true because Angelo was a very straightforward little boy and also because he'd heard stories from colleagues and patients that offered evidence that some children could remember events from inside the womb.

For example, our patient Kelsey shared an interaction with us that she'd had with her daughter, whom Shawn had delivered eight years earlier. She said:

For the longest time my daughter would describe a warm, comfortable kitchen she remembered from somewhere. It really bothered her that she couldn't remember whose kitchen it was or when she was there, but she felt like she had been there many times. One day while we were looking at photos, she grabbed one and exclaimed, "Mommy, this is it, this is the kitchen!" She was beaming from ear to ear.

It turned out that the kitchen Kelsey's daughter remembered was from the house where Kelsey had lived while she was pregnant. Kelsey said she loved to bake and truly loved that kitchen and all the delicious aromas and wonderful foods she was creating. She feels that her joy from that time period imprinted itself on her daughter, although she has no idea how her daughter was able to recount the designs and decorations of the kitchen.

 . . . .

Journaling Cue: Mentally relive the nine months of your pregnancy as if you are watching a movie on fast-forward. Feel free to hit the pause button along the way. Write down the events or circumstances when you were blissful, filled with joy and contentment. Note where you were at the time. Also write down the times you felt stressed out, angry, frightened, or frustrated. Why were you upset? Where were you at these times? Making an abbreviated record of your emotional highs and lows may help your child to someday connect important dots for their own spiritual or healing journeys.

Retrieval and Remedy of
Prenatal and Birth Memories

While we suspect that everyone has some memories from the time spent in utero, since not many people can place the memory as Kelsey's daughter was able to do, the memory eventually fades to the deeper recesses of our minds. And since the potential to retrieve these memories is compelling, there has been quite a lot of inquiry and research aimed at bringing the memory from the unconscious into the conscious. As intriguing as this information can be, many doctors and healers also acknowledge the impact that unearthing memories can have on people and the need for some type of supportive therapy.

Doctors Stan and Christina Grof integrated breathwork, evocative music, bodywork, and expressive arts into a therapy that has guided many participants back to their births. Their therapy, trademarked as Holotropic Breathwork, is a process that is intended to move the patient or client toward wholeness (thus the name holotropic). While there are reportable physical and psychological effects from this process, many participants reported memories from their own births from this type of therapy.

Participants experiencing perinatal memories simulate the physical and emotional aspects of being in the womb or of being born. And some patients are able to verify their memories through their own birth records. This type of therapy can be useful, not just for memory retrieval but to address symptoms such as headaches. Many people with chronic migraines credit this therapy with being the doorway to healing. They report that during this therapeutic process they felt themselves pushing through the birth canal or felt the doctor placing forceps on their heads. They describe rotation, pulling, and pain sensations, and some have gone back through their delivery records and verified they were delivered by forceps when this was unknown to them prior to the Holotropic Breathwork. In his book *The Holotropic Mind,* Grof describes the regression to birth as a four-tiered process through his interactions with patients:

The Amniotic Universe: Feelings of bliss and contentment as the participants claim these are the only feelings they are aware of. They feel protected, secure, and loved.

Cosmic Engulfment: No exit—the beginning of labor or that time of insecurity when the environment is shifting toward labor. There is a feeling of being stuck in a place that is chaotic and a sensation that there is no way out.

Death vs. Rebirth Struggle: The second stage of labor or when the mother is pushing. A struggle of survival in the sense that there is an impending change and shifting to being outside in an unknown world, leaving behind the security that one has known since formation. A metaphor for many changes in our lives, including death.

Death vs. Rebirth Experience: The birth of the baby. There is intense fear and chaos once again until the baby is placed with the mother, whom they recognize by voice and the intense joy and happiness of a new phase that begins with breastfeeding and continued bonding of the maternal-baby unit. Obviously this can be severely disrupted in those institutions where mother and baby are separated after birth, and Holotropic Breathwork participants have described this phenomenon.

Critics of Holotropic Breathwork say that the hyperventilation used to achieve an altered state of mind may cause seizures or other problems such as increased blood pressure and should only be undertaken if cleared by a medical practitioner. That being stated, this type of treatment is always to be done with a person who is responsible for guiding the patient when they begin to have the holotropic or transpersonal experience.

Rebirthing breathwork is a treatment that grew out of the work of New Thought philosopher Leonard Orr. Orr developed his theory after becoming a born-again Christian and spending hours and hours in the bathtub. He began having memories of time spent in the womb and being born.

Early participants would submerge themselves facedown in the bathtub and use a snorkel for breathing. Orr discovered there was a certain breathing pattern that occurred in most individuals and used this breathing pattern outside of the tub as the basis for his rebirthing breathwork. Along with Grof, Orr believed that the human birth process was and is a traumatic event, and that newborns suppress memories that later come out as different pathologies in adult life, like the chronic migraines of the man who retrieved the memory of being delivered by forceps. This doesn't suggest that forceps delivery causes headaches but rather that we can develop the headaches as physical manifestations of a traumatic memory. As of yet, there are no well-controlled studies of either of these techniques. However, the validity of breathwork in psychological cases has been examined and found to be beneficial as a therapeutic modality.[63]

Journeywork
On the Inside Looking Out

Holotropic Breathwork should be done with qualified professionals, so we can't give you a "do it yourself" journeywork for this experience. But we can offer you the opportunity to create a bridge to your subconscious memories by using your imagination.

Close your eyes, balance your breathing, and imagine you can see a large screen, as if you are seated in a movie theatre. See an image of yourself at age ten or so on the screen, then see an image of yourself as a toddler. Feel your attention turning inward as the screen shows a photograph of you as a newborn.

Take a few deep breaths and then imagine that you are this baby. You feel warm and safe, and you are inside your mother's belly. What does it feel like? What can you see? Do you hear anything? Follow this imagined scene and see what your mind suggests. When you open your eyes, write down everything you experienced.

By consciously reaching toward the subconscious, some of your dreams and daydreams may begin to include images that give you clues and open doorways to memories of your mother's womb.

Naturally, not all children talk about pre-birth memories, but we don't know if that's because not all children have these memories of if children have the memories but don't know how to share what they recall. It's possible that they don't even realize that these memories would be significant to the rest of us. Whatever the case, the important thing is to be receptive to whatever your child shares. Even if it sounds outrageous, resist the urge to cross-examine and instead gently inquire. There's no harm in hearing your child out, and who knows? You may learn something that amazes you.

Afterword

As One Journey Ends, Another Begins

You did it! You brought forth new life and deepened your connection with your soul, the your child's soul, and the world soul. You have completed a heroic, epic journey, transforming yourself along the way. Your courage and strength have been tested, and you have passed these tests with flying colors, some more easily than others. You have endured all manner of discomfort, walked through the fire of your anxieties and fears, and surrendered to the raw pain of childbirth, opening to the ecstasy of the miracle.

Today you stand in your power before God and Goddess with the understanding that you are strong, brave, and wise. You know that there is much to learn, but you also know that you're capable of meeting whatever challenges you encounter on the road ahead. As you traverse this path, you will be blessed with the connections you make with other mothers and the wisdom of all mothers who came before you. But the voice of your own soul will continue to be your wisest guide, just as it was during this epic journey. The more you continue to connect with the love and guidance of your soul, the easier it will be to tune in to the insights, inspiration, and ideas your soul has to share.

You now know, without a doubt, that this journey was as much about your transformation to motherhood as it was about being pregnant and giving birth. The journeywork you did opened gateways to new ways of seeing, sensing, and living. You, more than anyone, know how deeply this journey has changed you and how it's prepared you for the new journey of nurturing and guiding your child.

As you and your baby engage with the "ordinary world," be gentle with yourself and with your newborn. Transitions take time, and even though you know each other well on a soul level, there is much to be learned about navigating the physical world and building a life together. Resist the urge to be a "supermom" and instead be the best mom you can be for this particular child. The adage that it takes a village to raise a child is perhaps one of the most truthful statements about child development. Let go of the notion that you should do it all yourself. Gift your family members and loved ones with the opportunity to attend to the baby and to support you as you heal and acclimate to active motherhood.

Soon you will feel fully awake, alive, and well again. It may take a while before you're ready to be sexually active with your partner, and that's normal. Honor the love union that brought this new baby into your lives by sharing your love with your kindness, words, cuddling, and hugs until the time is right for more.

Just as you accepted the call to transformation at the onset of your pregnancy, you are now accepting the call to motherhood. During this adventure you will learn new ways to bond with your baby, your mate, and your other children. The mother-mentors who supported your pregnancy journey will now offer emotional and spiritual support in raising your new child. We encourage you to begin a new journey book to capture this joy, wonder, and bliss and to reflect on the trials and tribulations. And we highly recommend that you continue practicing the meditations, yoga poses, and relaxation and breathing exercises that you've learned. Being strong and flexible—mentally, physically, and spiritually—will empower you to greet each new day with confidence, an open mind, and an open heart.

Be attuned to your baby's vibrations, and when she begins to talk, listen carefully. She may reveal some pearls of wisdom or even share insights from the spirit realm. Just as some children recall their time in utero, some children recall the time before they were born. Your young child may have a message for you from one of your ancestors or wisdom to share. According to Annie Kagan, author of *The Afterlife of Billy Fingers: How My Bad-Boy Brother Proved to Me There's Life After Death*, we experience what might be called spiritual amnesia when we're born. From the afterlife, Billy told Annie, "When you're born, when you pop out, that big pop gives you a kind of amnesia. One of the main things we're doing when we're alive is trying to remember the things we forgot." For some children, some of the memories of life before birth are still intact. Billy also said, "Before each soul comes to earth, its own personal edition of the *Book of Life* is written." So if your child begins to share spiritual ideas or stories with you, we hope you will record these in his journey book so he can read them when he's older.

Your Motherhood Journey

The initiation stage of your new journey is ongoing as you and your child continually adjust to each other's growth and development. You will approach the inmost cave again when your child begins to make the transformation from childhood to adolescence. There's a reason we have thirteen or fourteen years to prepare for this stage of the journey! But just as you were ready to give birth at the close of your pregnancy journey, you will be ready to guide your child through the canal between childhood and adolescence when the time comes.

On your motherhood journey, the Holy Grail represents the full-grown adult whom you will have raised. At this point, you will have fulfilled your spiritual contract to prepare him for the world, and he will now venture out for his own hero's journey. But no matter how far he travels, your spiritual bond will beat between your hearts and light up your souls.

Blessed be.

Endnotes

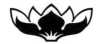

1 Robin Lim, www.facebook.com/robinlimbali?sk=
   wall&filter=1, December 16, 2011, Facebook wall.

2 Barbara Katz Rothman, www.barbarakatzrothman.com,
   December 16, 2012, website banner.

3 Andrea O'Reilly, *Encyclopedia of Motherhood* (California:
   Sage Publications Inc., 2010).

4 Bollingen Foundation. *The Hero with a Thousand Faces*
   (New York: MJF Books, 1949).

5 Rick Strassman, *DMT: The Spirit Molecule; A Doctor's
   Revolutionary Research into the Biology of Near-Death
   and Mystical Experiences* (Maine: Park Street Press,
   2001).

6 Ibid.

7 Joseph Campbell, *The Hero with a Thousand Faces*
   (California: New World Library, 2008).

8 Charles Spencer King, *Nature's Ancient Religion: Orisha
   Worship & IFA* (CreateSpace Independent Publishing,
   2008).

9   Mary Ellen Miller and Karl Taube, *An Illustrated Dictionary of the Gods and Symbols of Ancient Mexico and the Maya* (New York: Thames and Hudson, 1997).

10 Beatrice Fontanel and Claire d'Harcourt, *Babies: History, Art, and Folklore* (New York: Harry N. Abrams, 1997).

11 Ibid.

12 Ibid.

13 Ibid.

14 Ibid.

15 "Mother's Stress Harms Foetus," *Guardian*; www.guardian.co.uk, May 30, 2007, p. 2.

16 Mulder, E. J., et al. "Prenatal Maternal Stress: Effects on the Pregnancy and the (Unborn) Child," *Early Human Development* 70 (2002):3–14.

17 *Clin Endocrinol* (Oxf) 66, no. 5 (May 2007):636–40.

18 C. Sorgen, "Bonding with Baby Before Birth," WebMD, http://www.webmd.com/baby/features/ bonding-with-baby-before-birth, January 21, 2013.

19 T. Varney, *The Secret Life of the Unborn Child: How You Can Prepare Your Baby for a Happy, Healthy Life* (New York: Dell, 1982).

20 Olivia Lim and Sophia, "Prenatal Stimulation for a Smart Baby," Brainy Child, http://www.brainy-child .com/article/prenatal-stimulation.shtml, January 21, 2013.

21 D. Querleu et al., "Reaction of the Newborn Infant Less Than 2 Hours After Birth to the Maternal Voice," *Gynecol Obstet Biol Reprod* 13(2):125–34. PubMed .gov, http://www.ncbi.nlm.nih.gov/pubmed/ 6736589, January 21, 2013.

22 W. P. Fifer and C. M. Moon, "The Role of Mother's Voice in the Organization of Brain Function in the Newborn," *Acta Pediatrica* 83 (2008):86–93.

23 B. S. Kisilebvsky, et al., "Fetal Sensitivity to Properties of Maternal Speech and Language," Infant Behavior and Development (website), http://www.kangleelab .com/articles/Paper0001_0004_0001_0001.pdf, January 21, 2013.

24 Jo Harris, *Bonding Before Birth*. Website: birth.com.au, http://www.birth.com.au/Pregnancy/Pregnancy-29- 40-weeks/Emotions-during-the-last-three-months-of- pregnancy/Communicating-with-your-unborn-baby- how-to-bond-w, January 21, 2013.

25 J. Mennella, A. Johnson, and G. Beauchamp, "Garlic Ingestion by Pregnant Women Alters the Odor of Amniotic Fluid," *Chem Senses* 2 (Apr 20):207–9. Available at PubMed.gov, http://www.ncbi.nlm.nih .gov/pubmed/7583013.

26 Joseph Mercola, "Unplug! Too Much Light at Night May Lead to Depression," http://articles.mercola .com/sites/articles/archive/2012/08/09/too-much- night-light-causes-depression.aspx, December 15, 2012.

27 Barbara Kisilevsky, *Psychological Science* 2003, p. 650.

28   Luke 1:42, *Holy Bible, New International Version* (Maine: Zondervan Bibles, 2011).

29   The Humane Society of the United States, "Pregnancy and Toxoplasmosis," http://www.humanesociety.org/animals/resources/tips/toxoplasmosis.html, November 7, 2012.

30   Andrew Harvey, *Light upon Light, Inspirations from Rumi* (California: North Atlantic Books, 1996).

31   Karen Kingston, *Creating Sacred Space with Feng Shui* (New York: Broadway Books, 1997).

32   B. S. Kisilevsky, et al., "Maturation of Fetal Responses to Music," *Developmental Science 7*, Issue 5 (November 2004):550–59. Abrams et al. Donald J. Shetler (1985). Phyllis Evelyn Wilkin et al (1993). Eduardo de la Fuente at al (1997).

33   C. Vargas Dinicu, "Belly Dancing and Childbirth," *Sexology Magazine* 1964.

34   W. Buonaventura, *Serpent of the Nile* (MA: Interlink Books, 1989).

35   M. Cheyney, "Reinscribing the Birthing Body: Home Birth as Ritual Performance," *Medical Anthropology Quarterly* 4 (Dec. 25):519–42. Available October 22, 2012, at http://www.ncbi.nlm.nih.gov/pubmed/22338293

36   K. Modjarrad, "Medicine and Spirituality," *JAMA* 291 (2004):2880.

37   P. Ravenscroft and E. Ravenscroft, "Spirituality and Surgery," in G. P. Dunn and A. G. Johnson,

eds., *Surgical Palliative Care* (Oxford, UK: Oxford University Press; 2004), 65–84.

38 M. B. Råholm, "Weaving the Fabric of Spirituality as Experienced by Patients Who Have Undergone a Coronary Bypass Surgery," *J Holist Nurs.* 20 (2002):31–47.

39 American Medical Association, "Informed Consent," http://www.ama-assn.org/ama/pub/physician -resources/legal-topics/patient-physician-relationship- topics/informed-consent.page. October 1, 2011.

40 T. J. Kaptchuk, "The Placebo Effect in Alternative Medicine: Can the Performance of a Healing Ritual Have Clinical Significance?" *Ann Intern Med.* 136 (2002):817–25.

41 J. B. Moseley, K. O'Malley, N. J. Petersen, et al., "A Controlled Trial of Arthroscopic Surgery for Osteoarthritis of the Knee," *N Engl J Med.* 347 (2002):81–88.

42 C. S. Grob, "The Psychology of Ayahuasca," in R. Metzner, ed., *Sacred Vine of Spirits: Ayahuasca* (Rochester, VT: Park Street Press, 2006), 63–94.

43 M. Buber, *I and Thou* (W. Kaufmann, trans.), first Touchstone ed. (New York, NY: Free Press, 1971).

44 B. R. Kracht, "Kiowa Powwows: Continuity in Ritual Practice," *Am Indian Q* 18 (1994):321–48.

45 T. Csordas, *The Sacred Self: A Cultural Phenomenology of Charismatic Healing* (Los Angeles, CA: University of California Press, 1994).

46 L. Marks, "Sacred Practices in Highly Religious Families: Christian, Jewish, Mormon, and Muslim Perspectives," *Fam Process* 43 (2004):217–31.

47 M. Brady, S. Kinn, and P. Stuart, "Preoperative Fasting for Adults to Prevent Perioperative Complications," *Cochrane Database Syst Rev* 4 (2003):CD004423.

48 J. C. Rossiter and B. M. Yam. "Breastfeeding: How Could It Be Enhanced? The Perceptions of Vietnamese Women in Sydney, Australia," *J of Midwifery and Women's Health* 45 (2000):271–76.

49 V. Turner, *The Ritual Process: Structure and Anti-Structure* (Piscataway, NJ: Aldine Transaction, 1995).

50 L. M. Van Blerkom, "Clown Doctors: Shaman Healers of Western Medicine," *Med Anthropol Q* 9 (1995):462–75.

51 J. Endredy, *Lightning in My Blood: A Journey into Shamanic Healing and the Supernatural* (Woodbury, MN: Llewellyn, 2011).

52 S. J. Thomas, "The Sioux Medicine Bundle," *Am Anthropol* 43 (1941):605–9.

53 A. A. Gawande, D. M. Studdert, E. J. Orav, T. A. Brennan, and M. J. Zinner. "Risk Factors for Retained Instruments and Sponges After Surgery," *N Engl J Med* 348 (2003):229–35.

54 The archive for research in archetypal symbols (ARAS). Blue. In A. Ronnberg and K. Martin, eds., *The Book of Symbols* (Los Angeles, CA: Taschen, 2010).

55 C. B. Zhong and K. Lilienquist. "Washing Away Your Sins: Threatened Morality and Physical Cleansing," *Science* 313 (2006):1451–52.

56 A. Backster, A. Teo, M. Swift, H. C. Polk, and A. H. Harken, "Transforming the Surgical 'Time-Out' into a Comprehensive 'Preparatory Pause,'" *J Card Surg* 22 (2007):410–16.

57 The archive for research in archetypal symbols (ARAS). Wound. In A. Ronnberg and K. Martin, eds., *The Book of Symbols* (Los Angeles, CA: Taschen, 2010).

58 *Nurs.* 20 (2002):31–47. M. Eliade, *Shamanism: Archaic Techniques of Ecstasy* (New York: Pantheon Books, 1964).

59 S. A. Tassone, "Medical Materialism, Shamanic Healing, and the Allopathic Paradigm," http://www .realitysandwich.com/blog/7396, January 29, 2009.

60 B. G. Moynihan, "The Ritual of a Surgical Operation," *Br J Surg* 8 (1920):27–35.

61 C. A. Tanner, P. Benner, C. Chesla, and D. R. Gordon, "The Phenomenology of Knowing the Patient," *Image J Nurs Sch* 25 (1993):273–80.

62 J. Gilmartin and K. Wright, "Day Surgery: Patients Felt Abandoned During the Preoperative Wait," *J Clin Nurs* 17 (2008):2418–25.

63 J. S. Young and C. S. Cashwell, "Religion, Spirituality, and Supervision," in J. Culbreth and L. Brown, eds., *State of the Art in Clinical Supervision* (New York: Taylor Francis Routledge, 2010), 151–72.

Recommended Reading

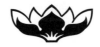

Creating Sacred Space with Feng Shui by Karen Kingston

The Hero with a Thousand Faces by Joseph Campbell

The Spirit Molecule: A Doctor's Revolutionary Research into the Biology of Near-Death and Mystical Experiences by Rick Strassman, M.D.

The Secret Life of the Unborn Child: How You Can Prepare Your Baby for a Happy, Healthy Life by Thomas Varney

Babies: History, Art, and Folklore by Beatrice Fontanel and Claire d'Harcourt

Shamanism: Archaic Techniques of Ecstasy by Mircea Eliade

Lightning in My Blood: A Journey into Shamanic Healing and the Supernatural by James Endredy

I and Thou (W. Kaufmann, trans.) by Martin Buber

Creating Sacred Space with Feng Shui by Karen Kingston

Light upon Light: Inspirations from Rumi by Andrew Harvey

Appendix A

Pregnancy Heals Your Spirit
by Pandora Peoples

Pregnancy is healing for the spirit. At this time you are a power-house. The purity, light, and love that your baby exudes from within is a direct connection with the Divine. As you direct love toward your belly and your womb, you are reconnecting with your body and a deeper ability to nurture yourself. Mother's intuition begins here as your consciousness expands with the synergy created between you and your child.

Your baby is receiving messages about your environment through fluctuations in your hormones, heartbeat, and voice as he acclimates to your emotional landscape from the inside. All of the stressors and stimulation surrounding you affect your baby, including the television programs you watch, the music you listen to, the conversations you have, and the exercise you do. The roller coaster of physical changes—including nausea, euphoria, mood swings, heartburn, increased libido, and discomfort during sleep—give you the opportunity to face each new sensation without fear or judgment. Living in the moment is a skill that behooves you in childbirth, so you can reject negative storylines and actively create the birth experience you desire. The fulfillment you get from an empowered pregnancy rewrites cultural mythologies of misery and pain passed from generation to generation. When we resist retreating to a fearful place, we respect the life emerging from us by offering unlimited opportunities to experience comfort, joy, and stability.

During my pregnancy, students at a birth class were asked to visualize and draw their babies. I sketched a boy in the womb with strong muscular legs, lean arms, and long eyelashes, next to an enormous purple-red placenta. Outside of the amniotic sac, I drew the protective hand of Archangel Michael. While giving birth, during transition, a huge wave of relief overcame me. Someone seemed to put a cool washcloth on my forehead. Suddenly, I felt safe and protected. I opened my eyes to see who was helping me, but my birth attendants were in another room. Was it Archangel Michael? Was my illustration a premonition or had it evoked the presence of the angel? At that moment, a surge of confidence from deep within took me into the active phase of labor.

My son was born lean, unusually muscular, with long, thick eyelashes. My husband still talks about how uncanny it is that the picture I drew resembled our son at birth. When I saw that our son's placenta was almost as big as he was, I knew that I had tapped into some significant truths in my drawing. It is such a beautiful souvenir to have from that time. The validation that came with drawing it helped me to have more faith in my intuition regarding my child.

Spiritual Pregnancy connects female wisdom to the lore of Grandmother Spider, personified as the creator of the universe in Native American cultures. The spider as an animal totem is also associated with weaving and women's wisdom. In my practice as a medium and intuitive healer, I have come to expound on this tradition of Grandmother's web responsible for birthing life into the universe outside the purely metaphysical realm. The World Wide Web is a series of electronic messages continually sent between people all over the globe. These energy exchanges have increased significantly as more people use portable devices to communicate via the Internet. The World Wide Web is a physical manifestation of the energetic interconnectedness all people innately share, which reflects the spiritual truth that we are each parts of a larger whole. The shared consciousness we possess is emerging in the contents of the Internet, wherein our collective knowledge and communal beliefs, ideologies, and perspectives converge en masse.

Most people know what it feels like to think someone is staring at them, only to turn around and see that they are indeed correct. Many people have had the experience of knowing who is calling before they see the number listed on the phone. And people often have experienced a telepathic connection with their children, best friend, or lover at one time or another. Have you ever known what someone was going to say before they said it or finished someone's sentence? These experiences are all indicative of the psychic link we share, and they hint at what we are capable of enjoying more often. With the advent of instant messaging, we are coming closer to understanding the way that Spirit communicates through energy directly and instantaneously. Feelings are the driving energetic force behind thoughts, and we can feel those from across a crowded room.

In the tradition of mediums, dating back thousands of years and spanning all cultures, people have understood the process of translating ideas and feelings from Spirit and those who have passed on. Through the work I do with my clients, I have come to understand that babies in the womb, although not communicating verbally, convey messages to their mothers that can be heard loud and clear. Pregnancy gives us tremendous opportunities to have faith in our own perceptions. The closeness shared between mother and child during this time is so intimate. Go ahead, treasure these expansive feelings of motherly love. Let it fill you up and invigorate you. Some moms become fearful of losing their babies and stave off celebrating until their babies are safely in their arms, yet it is prenatal bonding that gives us confidence in the birth process.

Belly Dancing

As mentioned in *Spiritual Pregnancy*, belly dance is the first documented form of dance, which evolved to instruct women in the preparation for childbirth. I began belly dancing four years after giving birth to my son, and it heralded a remarkable transformation from within. Not only does the bodywork help to turn off the mind, decreasing stress, but it also begins a process of deep healing and discovery. Movements help strengthen the pelvic floor, the Kegel muscles, and tone the perineum and abdomen, readying women for birth. Belly dance is also a perfect postpartum healing tool. It strengthens the pelvic floor and tones the vaginal walls, helping the uterus and associated muscles to return to their pre-pregnancy state. In my clients, I have seen it resolve uterine incontinence and increase core strength, with increased boosts of self-esteem and willpower.

The dance includes hip shimmies, which are the foundation to which you add belly rolls, chest lifts, head circles, arm waves, and finger movements. It is the ultimate in multitasking, making it the perfect tool to help women step into their superpowers. Any mother of a new baby knows the work she does can only be the work of a superhero.

Belly dance provides a safe way to express feminine sensuality and to recharge your body. The undulation of the spine seen in African and Middle Eastern dance stimulates all of the energy centers of the body, known in traditional Ayurvedic medicine as chakras. It is this movement that creates euphoria and ecstatic sensations described by orgasmic birthers. By improving your physical coordination while your pleasure center is stimulated, pathways in your brain make positive associations with multitasking, preparing you for all of the emotional, mental, and spiritual work being a mother entails.

Spiritual Clearing

People tend to compartmentalize aspects of themselves, as if they are looking at their to-do lists as scripts for their lives. *Time for work: check. Time for the kids: check. Date night: check. Spiritual retreat next year? Booked!* Although some compartmentalization is necessary, integrating our many aspects is what makes us cohesive, consistent, and effective parents. The sacred path we walk along is not a road we touch down on every now and then when we are centered enough to pay attention to our spiritual needs; it's the way we exist in our everyday lives. Pregnancy is a magical time that cultivates this connection. It offers us the opportunity to be more fully in our bodies and in the present moment.

The spiritual clearing ideas offered in this book for preparing your environment are a great way to let your nesting instincts kick in. In addition, a personal spiritual clearing has proven to be tremendously effective for my clients. Prepare for birth by purging old attitudes, beliefs, or fears that could work at cross-purposes to the fulfillment of your birth plan or that could negatively affect your parenting. This is a time for shedding layers of ego, or personality, that you have outgrown. A method I discovered is a modern-day rite of passage ritual.

During my pregnancy, some of my unrealized goals, regrets, and insecurities came up for me. A strong hunch led me to believe that if I did not let these go, my unconscious baggage would be in the driver's seat and lead me to confront my "stuff" in a dramatic way during birth. I really wanted my son's birth to be about him, and I wanted to address my issues head-on before his due date. I wanted resolve in every area of my life that I had experienced a struggle in, so that I could step into being a more confident, actively creative and empowered force in preparing myself for the initiation of birth.

Fortuitously, at that time my mother approached me with nine crates of my papers she was ready to release from her storage space. At first I railed against the timing: I was overwhelmed with preparations and work; I was deep cleaning, reclaiming the walls with no-VOC latex paint, buying baby supplies, building furniture, attending birthing classes, squeezing in prenatal exercises, chronicling my meals, Kegeling in the car, and seeing my clients. During a meditation at the beach, it dawned on me that this was my mother's unconscious way of supporting me in my need to shed my baggage, clear my head, and step into the role of mother. Instead of feeling overwhelmed or hurt that she no longer wanted to be responsible for my stuff, it gave me the opportunity for spiritual clearing. My mother was passing me the mother torch!

A rite of passage ritual for personal spiritual clearing may begin by gathering a handful of letters, memorabilia, photos, or other items that have unpleasant memories attached to them. Keeping such artifacts to remind you of the obstacles you have overcome or the victimization that you have endured only gives power to stories you may be tempted to repeat. Once patterns are established, they are woven into the fabric of your personal mythologies. These items should be either ceremoniously discarded or burned in a fire pit (be careful not to inhale the smoke). Let any evidence of suffering, haunting words, or negative thoughts fly free. Place the ashes into a houseplant or outdoor soil from which new growth can symbolically emerge. Thank Spirit for your blessings. It takes too much mental power to fit contrary evidence into a paradigm of outdated beliefs. Ask for support from Spirit, angels, or ancestors in letting go of what you want to leave behind as you enter this phase of new motherhood.

It turns out that being a portal from which new life emerges is a really big deal. Thankfully, the experience does prepare us for the challenges, bliss, and all-consuming involvement that being a mother requires from us. Most of all, it teaches us to be present with our selves and our babies. The preliminary work we do during pregnancy is integral to making childbirth easier. By connecting with our babies, toning our uterine muscles and perineum with bodywork, and clearing our spaces, we tap in to an intelligence that will guide us in childbirth.

My son's birth taught me that I could go from a profoundly uncomfortable place to an ecstatic and euphoric place in a matter of seconds. Before the crowning of my son's head, a shift took place within as I began rocking my pelvis back and forth, arching my spine, and kissing my husband. The last part of the birth had some profoundly sensual moments. It only makes sense to bring your baby into the world in the same way he was conceived: with love and pleasure.

Pandora Peoples is a psychic medium, herbalist, and writer offering workshops on connecting with the sacred feminine, healing with plants, and connecting with your guardian angels. To learn more about Pandora Peoples, visit her website at pandorasgarden.net.

Appendix B

A Journey of Firsts[*]
by Barbara Barnett

A woman of valor, who can find?
Far beyond rubies is her value...
She is like a merchant's ships; from
afar she brings her sustenance...
She rises while it is still nighttime,
and gives food to her household
and a ration to her maids.
She considers a field and buys it;
from the fruit of her handiwork
she plants a vineyard...
She girds her loins with might
and strengthens her arms.
Strength and splendor
are her clothing...
She opens her mouth with wisdom,
and the teaching of kindness is on her
tongue. She anticipates the needs of her
household, and the bread of idleness
she does not eat.
Her children rise and celebrate her;
and her husband, he praises her:
"Many daughters have attained valor,
but you have surpassed them all."
Excerpted from Proverbs 31:10–31

* Portions of this article appear in chapter 9.

Who is this impossible superwoman, this larger-than-life heroine-goddess described by the biblical Book of Proverbs? She seems to effortlessly straddle two worlds—spiritual and practical—and find balance in both. She is mother, wife, housekeeper, businesswoman, keeper of the family flame; she is idealized and impossible.

The previous nine months have been about you and the life growing inside you—an internal focus and preparation for the next leg of this amazing journey. This new journey has already begun; it began the moment you gave birth and gazed for the first time into your new baby's eyes.

The coming months will be a journey of firsts: first smile, first word, first step. The journey will be filled with wonder and amazement, but it will also be filled with challenges small and great.

During your pregnancy, you learned to understand the spiritual being within and place it in harmony with the new life that was growing inside you. It is possible to bring some of the divine, spiritual experience along with you as you enter into the ordinary rituals of parenting a newborn.

You might have imagined during your pregnancy what it would be like to bring home your newborn. If it is your first child, your imagination may have run wild with the idyllic, unhindered by experience (no matter what you might have been warned by friends and family).

Although you might have underestimated the challenges you now face, you also may have underestimated the incredible, the awesome, and the amazing. Finding the harmony between the two—finding balance between the challenges and the joy—is key to forging ahead on this next amazing journey. There will be moments you want to flee, to return to the beauty of dreams and imaginings, but there exists no retreat. This journey is yours to complete. Step back into your world—as you had known it; as it has changed—girded by the power you now contain within you.

As a new parent, you see the world through new eyes. So much has changed, even the mundane tasks of parenthood: bath time, nail cutting, and feeding can take on new meaning infused with a profound sense of awe.

The spiritual journey of pregnancy has changed the way you see things as you step back into your new life and onto your new path. It will allow you to find depth and beauty in the everyday and allow spirituality to infiltrate into the life around you, allowing your spirit to be touched by even the smallest thing. More than ever before, your life is now filled with "wow" moments. Allow yourself to experience them.

Your new baby is curious about everything she sees, hears, tastes, touches, and smells. Following his lead, learn to find the wow in what your baby senses. Let yourself experience her sense of wonder for yourself, putting you in tune with the world around you in a way that hasn't happened since you were a child yourself. It will enable you to connect with the Divine in ways you never imagined—and also put you in harmony with what your baby senses. What does he want to experience, see, and touch?

What is it that your baby sees that she finds so fascinating? Is it the colorful fish in your aquarium she's following with her eyes as they dart from one end to the other, or is it some subtler mystery that's attracted her attention? Perhaps it's the way the light glints off the coral or illuminates the ripples in the water. Maybe it's that scratch in the glass you haven't noticed in ages (if ever).

Wonder is to take wow a step further to something else. Wonder is a state of mind that allows us to look past memorized knowledge, enabling us to find the extraordinary in the ordinary and be amazed. It's to find that spark of the Divine in everything.

Twentieth-century philosopher Abraham Joshua Heschel wrote extensively about radical amazement. "Mankind will not perish for want of information," he said, "but only for want of appreciation." Allow yourself to ask the "why" behind each new wow moment. Can science explain it—or is there something indefinable and ineffable that can only be connected with the Divine?

Getting back to the light and how it plays on the scratch in your aquarium, you see that same light as it casts rainbows on your wall, glinting off a small scratch in the aquarium and its "wow." But its mystery goes deeper, into the source of light—of all light.

Can you take wonder even further, transcending the moment to explore what lies beyond this singular moment—when wonder becomes awe? Heschel defines awe as "the awareness of transcendent meaning, of a spiritual suggestiveness of reality (a sense that something lies behind and created the moment of wonder)."

It is, he said, an "answer of the heart and mind to the presence of mystery in all things, an intuition for a meaning that is beyond the mystery, an awareness of the transcendent worth of the universe." Let your new baby be your guide.

A Universe of Sensation

Your new baby not only uses his eyes to perceive the amazing world, each sense is put to use to discover and explore. You also use your senses to understand your child's needs, delights, and discomforts. Sounds, sensations, smells (not always so pleasant), and tastes take on greater meaning and connect you to your newborn's new world.

Every living thing has its own way of communicating. As a new parent you will soon be hearing with that special radar custom-tuned to your baby's unique frequency. You will know the crashing, resounding cymbals of his cries: tired, hungry, distressed, lonely—or in pain.

Although your baby's cries are sometimes enough to rattle your nerves, there are sounds that will be music to your ears. You will know the harp sounds of her contentment, his coos, her distinct laughter, the percussion of his sighs, her snores. Since your new child can't yet talk, you have to learn his language quickly; it is articulate and forceful—but possibly as strange to your ears as any foreign tongue. But you will learn to speak her language quickly enough!

But what does your newborn hear? Watch him as he responds to the sound of your voice. Listen to how she calms to the soothing lilt of your tone and giggles to the new sounds she experiences. Babies startle at unexpected noises, yelling, and chaos, but they love the sound of gentle music and the bounce of lively tunes. Sing to your child; babies are the most uncritical music critics in the world. Your voice will be divine and sublime.

Help your baby connect to the new world by introducing them to new sounds: a bird, the meow of your cat, the rush of a plane overhead as she becomes more accustomed to this new experience of hearing. Stop and listen for the melodies of your environment, perhaps as you never have before.

Touch

Babies love to touch. They find fascination with the angles and planes of faces, eyeglasses, noses—pretty much anything. Their tiny fingers reach out to explore and discover their new environment. They curl around your finger, they bat at your eyes, they feel your hair. What are they feeling? Is it the texture? The warmth? What are they trying to understand about this other being, soon to be known as Mommy or Daddy?

Touch is something adults usually take for granted, but tactile sensations can connect us to the spiritual and lead us to awe as profoundly as the things we see. The softness of a puppy as we stroke her fur and feel the downiness and warmth throughout our fingertips brings pleasure and provides comfort. The velvet of a rose's petals feels sublime on the fingers.

Then there is the feel of a baby—your new baby—cuddled close to you, warm and snug. It brings you pleasure, but the feeling is mutual. Touch, cradling, and cuddling are absolute necessities for both you and your baby. We all need to be touched, held, and cradled, even as adults.

Babies love and need to be touched; it's how they connect with the new humans in their lives—how they bond with you. Babies cannot be held and cuddled too much. In many cultures and for many centuries, swaddling has been a crucial part of making a newborn feel safe, secure, loved, and touched.

Of course the most intimate time for touching each other comes with feeding time. If you are nursing, you and your baby are connected physically with each other as she draws milk from your breast. It is miraculous that a baby's nourishment is provided; a perfect food, it is manna in liquid form.

If you are bottle-feeding, the connection is just as profound as you hold your child close to you, cuddled in the crook of your arm. You watch his face as he hungrily sucks, listen to her satisfied sigh when finished, the inevitable burp that lets you know he is comfortable and satiated.

Bath time also becomes an abundance of sensory riches. The act of washing the creases and folds of your baby's skin can become a source of amazement. Revel at the idea that this tiny person—this tiny "you"—grew for nine months inside you, your only inkling being a shadow on an ultrasound scan. And now here he is, sitting in the warm water as you gently clean him. Observe her toes: tiny and fragile, delicate nails—and so soft. Observe his legs that kicked and prodded for all those months, distending your abdomen as they poked from within. Now they are round and chubby, soft, with nearly translucent skin as you gently wash them.

Move up your baby's body and observe this little person whom you created in partnership with the Divine, a legacy that goes back to the beginning of time itself. You are connected through this baby to God, to your parents, and to the next segment of a sacred chain linking generation to generation. See her abdomen, the belly button—a prominent souvenir of her everlasting connection to you. Touch the softness of her downy skin, the fragile capillaries, blue just beneath the surface. Feel her heart beating, her arms splashing. Is she remembering her pre-birth home in the amniotic fluid of your belly?

Be amazed at her arms, her hands, his fingers—graceful in their grasping at anything and everything. Find wonder in his eyes, the softness of his hair, the bow of her lips.

Be amazed at this brilliant creation you have helped form!

Barbara Barnett serves large and small congregations as a cantor and ritual educator, guiding adults and children to find spiritual expression through Jewish prayer, text study, and song. She has written an award-winning parent-tot prayer book, as well as other publications for Jewish audiences, and speaks on spirituality, liturgy, and culture in front of audiences large and small, including Limmud Chicago.

Appendix C

Kabbalah and Creation
by Nina Amir

The Kabbalists, or Jewish mystics, say Creation happened when God, who was everywhere and everything, contracted to make space for something else to exist. Into the void created within Itself, God placed a beam of divine light. As it passed through the empty space in the womb of God's existence, something new that had never existed came into being.

When a woman conceives, in that moment an amazing, divine transformation begins in her "void." In the womb of her existence, something new comes into being—a human life.

The soul of that physical being, however, is not new. Each individual cycles through lives in what is known as *gilgul neshamot*, or soul cycle, reincarnating into different bodies at different times depending upon their particular task in the physical world, their spiritual level, and their part in creating and healing (*tikkun*) the world.

The mother and baby begin their spiritual journey together before conception. God realizes the time has come for a particular soul to enter a body and that a particular woman is the right mother for the child, and her partner the right father. They are chosen as the soul's parents whether they want to be or not or are ready to be or not. Thus, the ancient rabbis said each child has three parents: the mother, the father, and God.

A child travels from the heavenly realms into the physical world assisted through conception by an angel named Lailah, who first brings the soul before God. There the child's future is decided.

God then bids the soul to enter the embryo. The soul, who has been enjoying the bliss of its heavenly existence, takes on this task unwillingly, and then Lailah transports the child to the mother's womb.

There the embryo grows in a sacred space for nine months. And, indeed, the womb is a sacred space, for all Jewish women are *kohanot*, priestesses, with the awesome ability to create life, to determine the spiritual identity of their children, and to invoke the presence of the Shechinah, the Divine Feminine.

During the months when the soul transforms in the womb, it becomes the mother's job to influence the fetus's inner and outer environment. Jewish tradition encourages pregnant women to zealously guard their positive outlooks and perspectives by avoiding situations that bring them down emotionally, such as those that cause them anger or fear. All their emotions affect the growing child.

On a more spiritual level, the Kabbalists taught that pregnant women should involve themselves in *segulot*, or auspicious practices, used for hundreds, possibly thousands, of years to assist in bringing about a safe pregnancy and birth. Lighting Sabbath candles and giving to charity, or even taking a moment to offer gratitude for the gift of life, have ripple affects in both the physical and the spiritual worlds—and in the world of the developing child.

The ancient rabbis explain that a connection exists between a mother's spiritual state and the spiritual development of the fetus during pregnancy, before and during conception. The higher the mother's spiritual vibration, the higher that of the child's spiritual vibration, or spiritual state, when born and throughout life. The more spiritually educated the mother, the better she will be able to educate her child and support him in his spiritual journey. The story is told of a Jewish mother who approached a Torah sage and asked, "When should I begin the education of my child?"

"How old is your youngster?" he inquired.

"Five months old," she replied.

The sage pulled on his beard and shook his head. "You are already fourteen months too late."

In the womb the child is also receiving a private spiritual education to prepare for earthly existence. The sages say that the child lies in the dark fluids of the womb but with a view forward to her whole life and how the spiritual lessons she is learning can impact her life and her purpose for coming into the physical realm. Two angels teach her Torah and position a light above the baby's head, allowing her to see from one end of the world to the other. The child views all that she will experience in her life and is taught *mitzvot*, or how to live righteously and spiritually in the world. She learns that if she observes these rules, she will discover how to be close to God and fulfill her purpose. She realizes that this will give her life meaning, and she becomes ready for life—eager for life. She changes from a soul unwilling to take on a body to one unwilling to die.

Also while inside the sacred space, each morning an angel carries the child's spirit into Paradise, or the Garden of Eden, to see the righteous who lived a good life while in the physical world. In the evening the angel takes the child to hell, or Gehanna, to see how the wicked are punished after death.

Finally, when God determines the right time, the same angel who brought her into the womb orders the child to be born. At the moment of birth, the angel extinguishes the light above her head, and with a kiss on the upper lip that leaves an indentation (some say with a flick of a finger to the indentation of the lip) causes the child to forget every last thing she has seen and learned in the womb. Now begins the process of remembering, for all that learning remains present in the child's unconscious.

The baby does not need to be taught spiritual lessons and laws, only help in recalling them.

As the woman prepares to give birth, she feels the Shechinah settling down beside her, preparing to serve as her midwife. Out of the womb of her existence, something that has never existed before comes into existence. A new human life is born. And the *kohenet* reaches down and anoints him with oil upon his head and upon the bottom of his feet and on the palms of his hands and on the cleft of his lip. Like Adam in the Garden of Eden, she gives him a name.

. . . .

Nina Amir offers practical spiritual tools that span religious lines and are pertinent to people of all faiths and spiritual traditions. Amir is a certified rebirther and the author of seven books on practical spirituality, all with a foundation in Jewish mysticism but relevant to readers from all faiths. To learn more about Nina Amir, visit her website at www .ninaamir.com.

Appendix D

The Sukkah of Your Pregnancy
by Barbara Barnett

In the traditional Jewish prayer Hashkiveinu, we ask God to protect us from the things that go bump in the night—the monsters in the closet where the wild things dwell. It ends with a plea for God to cover us with a *sukkah*—a shelter—of peace. It's an extraordinary image. The sukkah is, by nature, temporary—enduring yet fragile—just strong enough to last through the week of the Sukkot festival or, allegorically, through the night.

It is a great metaphor for pregnancy. The uterus, like the sukkah, is fragile yet strong enough to protect the life growing within it. Temporary yet enduring; fragile, yet it's elastic enough to withstand tremendous stretching and absorb the constant kicks and other movements of the life growing within it. But more than that, the image of uterus-as-sukkah suggests a profound sense of the partnership with God in the constant cycle of creation. It is sacred space.

There is a Sukkot tradition of symbolically inviting biblical guests (*ushpizin*) into the sukkah: Sarah and Abraham, Rebecca and Isaac, Rachel, Leah, and Jacob, their spirits joining in for a little metaphorical home hospitality and perhaps to impart a little ancestral advice. What if we could transfer all that spiritual energy of the sukkah and those special guests to the sacred space surrounding pregnancy, not for a week, but for nine months?

Months One and Two

"When God began to create heaven and earth, the earth was unformed and void, with darkness over the surface of the deep and a the spirit of God sweeping over the water…" Can you imagine these opening words of the Torah (the Five Books of Moses) playing out in the microcosm of your body?

The first weeks when the chaos of a barely present amniotic sac might be imagined as an untranslatable Hebrew word, *tohu va'vohu*, that the Torah uses to describe the state of the universe on the first day of creation. The tohu va'vohu of the uterus divides and grows, just as the waters present during the seven days of Creation took shape as the heavens and the earth. The void is full of potential and energy just waiting to be expended.

"Let there be an expanse in the midst of the water, that it may separate water from water," says the Torah's text just a few verses later. As your pregnancy takes root within the uterus, you can only imagine, perhaps as you miss that first menstrual cycle and the first inklings of pregnancy begin to dance in your imagination, the beginning of the cell division and growth within—your own internal fluids separating, differentiating, creating during the first few weeks, before you can even sense the fetus.

"Let the water below the sky be gathered in one area, that the dry land may now appear." Visualize now your baby taking form in the midst of the womb's ocean—the formless taking shape—viable, tangible.

For the first two months you silently construct the sukkah of the womb, perhaps not even knowing it. Creating a baby is one of the wonders of nature, and if ever there is a profound sense that we are God's partners in the ongoing act of creation, it is upon learning of this new creation.

Imagine Eve, the first woman, watching over, keeping vigil from just outside the garden. Eve—the mother of us all, and the first woman—Adam's partner in the entire human enterprise. Adam and Eve were commanded to be fruitful and multiply. Although it was Eve who got Adam to take that infamous bite of the apple, we also can comprehend Eve to have had an amazing sense of wonder! It is her curiosity, her sense of newness in the human adventure that makes her a perfect first guest in your sukkah.

Month Three

The fact that you're pregnant is really settling in. Into your shiny new sukkah invite Sarah, the first Jewish mother—the mother of a nation. Sarah was a bold adventurer, journeying beside her husband to points unknown—a place of promise where their offspring would thrive. Their journey was not an easy one. Fraught with danger and the unknown, Sarah and Abraham eventually reached their destination to begin their family—their nation. But Sarah remained childless for many years before becoming a mother at the age of ninety! Sarah's reaction when she learned she was to be a mother? She laughed. "My husband is too old," she complained to God, falling on her face in peals of laughter, naming her son Isaac, which means laughter. So welcome Sarah, the prototypical Jewish mother, into your sukkah to help you find the humor and ironies of the weeks and months to come.

Month Four

Just as the sukkah inside you is getting bigger, so the sukkah surrounding you as you let more and more people into your intimate circle and let the news be known. It is a good month to welcome one of the bravest women from Jewish tradition, Queen Esther (also known as Hadasah). Esther was a brave young woman who saved an entire people by risking her life to plead for the lives of the Jews of Persia when confronted with possible annihilation. Although God's name is never mentioned in the biblical Book of Esther, God's Divine Presence, Shechinah, inhabits every line, hidden within the text and subtext. The name Esther itself may be translated as "concealment," and to some this suggests her ability to see beyond the obvious and find the Divine Presence where it hid, drawing strength from it—enough to save her people. Her other name, Hadassah, means "myrtle," one of the four species significant to Sukkot. The myrtle leaves represent human eyes and Esther's special insight—her ability to see beyond the obvious. Esther is the perfect guest to welcome during this month when so much is revealed—your pregnancy is harder and harder to conceal, and very little remains hidden to your friends, family, and colleagues. But it is also, in some ways, perhaps, a time of uncertainty and even anxiety. A little of Esther's courage is a good thing.

Month Five

During the fifth month you reach the halfway point, and perhaps you're now really beginning to feel like a mom. If you work outside the home, perhaps colleagues are beginning to wonder about your post-pregnancy plans even as you try to maintain your identity as a professional and keep your career afloat amid doctor visits, gentle jostlings from within, and your own changing physical and emotional state. The prophet Deborah was a judge in ancient Israel—a tribal leader, unusual for a woman of the time. When her people were threatened, she sent her general Barak to do battle, but he refused to go without this strong, intelligent, independent woman at his side. Deborah was much more than a military strategist and prophet. She was wife, mother, singer of songs, and weaver of verse. In the Book of Judges, she calls herself "a Mother in Israel," clearly a woman trying to reconcile the tension between professional responsibilities and nurturing maternal nature.

Month Six

Entering the final month of your second trimester, you are hopefully feeling great and not too tired. Your baby-to-be may be moving more and more, and you may even feel a few slight contractions as your body practices for the final show. Your pregnancy sukkah has expanded within you as you've gotten larger, but also the sukkah that surrounds you has also grown to accommodate family and friends who are just as excited as you are about the birth of your child. Among them may be an older, more experienced friend or family member who can prove to be a wise guide to accompany you the rest of the way, spiritually and in other ways as well.

The Book of Ruth is a love story. But it is also a story of a young woman who finds guidance and mentoring from an older woman. Widowed at a young age, a lonely and impoverished Ruth is told to return to her family by her mother-in-law Naomi. Instead, Ruth chooses to follow Naomi and acquires the friendship and guidance of a woman who had been through much in her lifetime. This month might be just the time to call on an older coworker, a close friend, your own mother-in-law or grandmother, or a cherished aunt who can give you practical advice and spiritual support in ways different than your partner or mother.

Month Seven

If this is your first child (or even your second or third), you may by now imagine what you will be like as a new mother. Will you be like your own—or will you find a different path to nurturing your children? How can you learn from your mother's successes and failures as you bring this new life to fruition? Perhaps you might understand more of what your own mother may have gone through—the physical, certainly, but also the emotional; draw spiritual energy from that unique connection.

For this reason, invite Moses' mother, Yocheved, into your pregnancy sukkah. In the Torah, Yocheved hid Moses to avoid the pharaoh's decree that all male Israelite children be killed upon birth. She represents the fiercely protective nature of mothers (and fathers) toward their children. Let her bring her nurturing and protective spirit into your sukkah.

Month Eight

Moses' sister Miriam's great gift was her well, which followed her throughout the wilderness, providing life-giving fresh water as the Israelites made their way from slavery to liberation. The life force of water surrounds your baby-to-be as she floats around, testing limbs, kicking, and sending waves rippling to the surface.

Miriam also represents the joyful dance and song of liberation, which she sang as the Israelites were born into a new state of being, no longer dependent on the tenuous umbilical cord of slavery.

Month Nine

Speaking of Miriam and Moses, the entirety of the Israelite deliverance from slavery to independence is a beautiful metaphor for the final stages of pregnancy and into labor and delivery, their forty-year journey into freedom symbolic of the forty weeks of pregnancy. The Israelites' journey began with two midwives, Shifra and Puah. Although ordered by the pharaoh to kill any male child born among the Israelites, they refused at great risk. They wouldn't harm the newborns, and their tenacity prevented an entire Israelite generation—the one that finally secured its freedom—from annihilation. Once finally liberated, the Israelites crossed the Red Sea, its waters parting. Imagine the birth canal—an image of a red sea of waters and blood parting and making way for your baby's head as it crowns. Closing again once its task is complete, the welcome cries of your baby, the song that Moses, Miriam, and all the children sang once they crossed to the other side—from attachment to independence, the cord severed. Manna, which came, according to the biblical text, from the heavens above, essentially the milk expressed from your full breasts. Complete nourishment in an elegant package—nothing more needed—the ultimate comfort food. There are no better guests to invite into these last weeks and days of your pregnancy sukkah than the midwives Shifra and Puah. Let them join Miriam, their contemporary out of the antiquity of Jewish history.

Barbara Barnett serves large and small congregations as a cantor and ritual educator, guiding adults and children to find spiritual expression through Jewish prayer, text study, and song. She has written an award-winning parent-tot prayer book, as well as other publications for Jewish audiences, and speaks on spirituality, liturgy, and culture in front of audiences large and small, including Limmud Chicago.

Appendix E

The Christian Mother
by Phoebe Collins

A Christian mother often has Mary in mind. The virgin birth of Jesus is a tenet of Christianity which holds that Mary miraculously conceived Jesus while remaining a virgin. This doctrine was a universally held belief in the Christian church by the second century A.D. and is maintained by Roman Catholicism, the Church of the East, Eastern Orthodoxy, Oriental Orthodoxy, Protestantism, and Anglicanism. While the spiritual image of Our Lady is most often associated with Roman Catholicism, Christians of all denominations recognize Mary as the earthly mother of Jesus Christ.

Mary's pregnancy began in the most unlikely, indeed frightening, way possible, with a late-night visit from an angel. This is called the Annunciation, and at first, the future mother of God questioned her role. She demanded of the heavenly apparition how she, a virgin, could possibly be pregnant. Mary is at first "greatly troubled." The preternatural words of the young Jewish peasant girl have come to be known as the Magnificat, or the Song of Mary. In it, she expresses her joy at being chosen to become a mother. Her joy arises despite difficult circumstances: her unmarried state, her extreme youth—all this pales beside rejoicing at the new life she has been chosen to bring forth.

It can be startling to those who are in happily committed relationships to think that God chose an unwed teenager to be the mother of his son. Hopefully, any expectant mother who finds herself in a challenging situation can look to Mary for inspiration and encouragement. Our own guardian angels may not be as forcefully present as Mary's, but unseen angels offer a source of strength and love when we choose to turn to them. For Mary, one conceptual worldview is replaced by another as she comes to terms with the true magnitude of what has happened to her, that the "mighty one" has done great things for her. After all, it's no small thing to consider that, in the times and culture that Mary lived in, pregnancy outside of wedlock was punishable by death.

Fortunately, Mary can see beyond her immediate surroundings. She envisions herself as part of a long chain of people stretching out backward to the past and forward to the future to include all of humanity. Ancestors are prominently remembered when she acknowledges God's promise to Abraham and his descendants. What ancestors will your baby take after? Whose eyes will you see in the little ones looking up at you for the first time? Take a look at yourself in the mirror or leaf through the photo album to see what physical resemblances occur in your own family. All these are the generations Mary referred to who will call her blessed. And, just as Mary can show us something about being human, your innocent little baby can show you something about what God is like—the God with whom Mary found great favor. A special prayer for pregnant Catholic and other Christian women asks for Mary's intercession at this most joyous yet sometimes tumultuous time:

> *Dearest Mary, I look to you now for the help of your maternal love. You understand my trials as an expectant mother. You bore Jesus in your womb. You know the doubts and anxieties that beset me; you know the bodily suffering I endure. Like you, may I turn all these sorrows into joy. You overcame anxiety by a loving trust in God; you overcame doubt by gentle resignation to His will. Your motherhood lifted your mind above earth and kept it close to God. So speak to Jesus now with me, beloved Mother, as I seek prayerfully to learn to bear the trials of motherhood with joy. Mother of Perpetual Help, pray for me!*

How does this affect a Christian mother's thoughts? The people she'll choose to serve as godparents take on special importance at such a time, as they supersede the usual requirements of relatives or close friends. She must choose people who will uphold the child's spiritual life and serve as role models, as well as special friends. Some questions she may ask herself regard the church-going habits of her friends and whether they are members of a congregation who take the Christian life seriously.

Once the baby is born, for Catholics the sacrament of baptism must take place one month after the baby's birth. This is not superstition, but rather a way of making sure the baby is welcomed into the worldwide Catholic communion as soon as possible. In the old days, early baptism was practiced in case the baby did not survive, as was too often the situation in the days before modern medicine. Interestingly, in an emergency of any kind, a priest is not necessary to perform the rite of baptism; any baptized Catholic will do. This is a highly unlikely circumstance, however, and a traditional baptism at the parents' parish, usually taking place during or after a regular Sunday mass, is the rule rather than the exception.

Baptism is the rite of welcome, celebration, and initiation for most Christian infants. Christians of practically all denominations believe that in baptism, babies are reborn through water and the Holy Spirit, and are cleansed of original sin. In passing through the water, Christians believe the baptized person shares in Jesus's death and resurrection. In Protestant denominations there is no rule for the time of the baby's baptism, or christening. While usually held in a church, the ceremony can also be performed at home amid family and friends, with a clergyperson presiding in an altogether more informal setting. Whatever the setting, a Christian mother will reach out in new ways to others, not just friends and family, but to God.

A favorite psalm is number 139:13–16: "For you created my inmost being; you knit me together in my mother's womb. I praise you because I am fearfully and wonderfully made; your works are wonderful, I know that full well. My frame was not hidden from you when I was made in the secret place, when I was woven together in the depths of the earth. Your eyes saw my unformed body; all the days ordained for me were written in your book before one of them came to be." The psalmist here affirms God's presence in virtually every aspect of our existence, from conception onward.

. . . .

As an acquisitions editor, Phoebe Collins has worked on a broad variety of books for the Catholic market. She also participates in the Los Angeles Religious Education Congress. Currently a consultant at Columbia University's Writing Center, her company, Exaudi Communications, focuses on Christian-themed projects of all kinds.

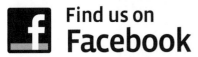
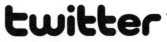
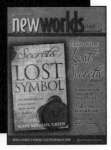

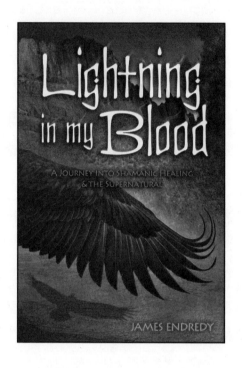

To order, call 1-877-NEW-WRLD

Prices subject to change without notice

Order at llewellyn.com 24 hours a day, 7 days a week!

Lightning in My Blood
A Journey into Shamanic Healing
& the Supernatural
James Endredy

James Endredy invites you on a wondrous journey into the shape-shifting, mind-altering, and healing magic of shamanism. For decades, Endredy has worked with wise tribal elders around the world, participating in their sacred ceremonies and learning from powerful animal guides and spirits. Here he relives these profound experiences, including his first meeting with a spirit guide that led to the seer's path, a terrifying lesson in using his ethereal body in the Sierra Madre mountains, how he outwitted an evil sorceress, and his incredible inauguration into shamanic healing.

Grouped by shamanic medicines, Endredy's captivating accounts highlight a fascinating tradition and the extraordinary journey of a modern shaman.

978-0-7387-2147-7
6 x 9 • 240 pp.

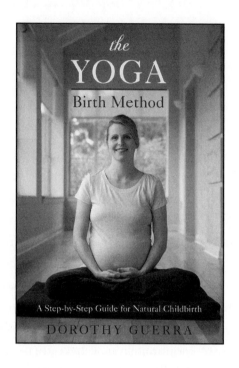

To order, call 1-877-NEW-WRLD

Prices subject to change without notice

Order at llewellyn.com 24 hours a day, 7 days a week!

The Yoga Birth Method
A Step-by-Step Guide for Natural Childbirth

Dorothy Guerra

Plan a childbirth that's calm, natural, and enlightened. *The Yoga Birth Method* is an empowering eight-step pathway to achieving a positive and joyful birth experience.

Applying the wisdom of yoga to childbirth, Dorothy Guerra offers a solid plan for managing the mind, body, and spirit throughout the stages of pregnancy and labor. Couples choose an intention that becomes a focal point for embracing a calm state of mind throughout the physical and emotional challenges of childbirth. You'll discover what to expect during each stage of labor and how to manage pain, eliminate anxiety, and encourage labor progression with breathing techniques and yoga poses. There's also guidance in drafting a birth plan, labor-support techniques for birth partners, information on medical intervention, and a "go to" chapter with checklists to use when the big day arrives.

978-0-7387-3665-5
6 x 9 • 240 pp.

To Write to the Authors

If you wish to contact the authors or would like more information about this book, please write to the authors in care of Llewellyn Worldwide and we will forward your request. Both the authors and the publisher appreciate hearing from you and learning of your enjoyment of this book and how it has helped you. Llewellyn Worldwide cannot guarantee that every letter written to the authors can be answered, but all will be forwarded. Please write to:

Shawn Tassone and Kathryn Landherr
℅ Llewellyn Worldwide
2143 Wooddale Drive
Woodbury, MN 55125-2989

Please enclose a self-addressed stamped envelope for reply
or $1.00 to cover costs. If outside the USA, enclose
an international postal reply coupon.

Many of Llewellyn's authors have websites with additional information and resources. For more information, please visit our website:

www.llewellyn.com